ABC OF
RESUSCITATION

Fifth Edition

ABC OF RESUSCITATION

Fifth Edition

Edited by

M C Colquhoun
Chairman of the Resuscitation Council (UK)

A J Handley
*Past chairman of the Resuscitation Council (UK) and Chairman of
ILCOR working party on basic life support*

and

T R Evans
Past chairman of the Resuscitation Council (UK)

BMJ
Books

© BMJ Publishing Group 2004

First edition 1986
Second edition 1990
Third edition 1995
Fourth edition 1999
This edition published in 2004
by BMJ Publishing Group, BMA House, Tavistock Square,
London WC1H 9JR

www.bmjbooks.com

British Library Cataloguing in Publication Data

A catalogue record for this book is available from the British Library

ISBN 0 72791669 6

Typeset by Newgen Imaging Systems (P) Ltd., Chennai, India
Printed and bound in Malaysia by Times Offset

Cover image shows a computer-enhanced image of an electrocardiogram trace showing showing an abnormal heart beat (red). A healthy heartbeat is seen at the top (yellow) for comparison with permission from Mehan Kulyk/Science Photo Library

Contents

Contributors

Peter J F Baskett
Consultant Anaesthetist Emeritus, Frenchay Hospital and the Royal Infirmary, Bristol

Bob Bingham
Consultant Anaesthetist, Great Ormond Street Hospital for Children NHS Trust, London

Ian Bullock
Head of Education and Training, Royal Brompton and Harefield NHS Trust; and Honorary Clinical Teaching Fellow, Imperial College, London

A John Camm
Professor of Clinical Cardiology, St George's Hospital Medical School, London

Douglas Chamberlain
Professor of Resuscitation Medicine, University of Wales College of Medicine, Cardiff

Michael Colquhoun
Senior Lecturer in Prehospital Care, Wales Heart Research Institute, Cardiff

C Sian Davies
Programme Manager, National Defibrillator Programme, the Department of Health, London

Charles D Deakin
Consultant Anaesthetist, Southampton University Hospital, Southampton

T R Evans
Consultant Cardiologist, Royal Free Hospital, London

Carl Gwinnutt
Consultant Anaesthetist, Hope Hospital, Salford

Anthony J Handley
Consultant Physician and Cardiologist, Colchester

Mark Harries
Consultant Physician, Northwick Park and St Mark's NHS Trust, Harrow

Roy Liddle
Resuscitation Training Officer, Wythenshaw Hospital, Manchester

Andrew K Marsden
Consultant Medical Director, Scottish Ambulance Service, Edinburgh

Anthony D Milner
Emetrius Professor of Neonatology, Guy's and St Thomas's Hospital Trust, London

Stephen Morris
Consultant Obstetric Anaesthetist, Llandough Hospital and Community NHS Trust, South Glamorgan

Jerry Nolan
Consultant Anaesthetist, Royal United Hospital, Bath

Peter A Oakley
Consultant in anaesthesia and trauma, Department of Trauma Research, University Hospital of North Staffordshire, Stoke on Trent

Gavin D Perkins
Research Fellow in Intensive Care Medicine, Birmingham Heartlands Hospital, Birmingham

David Pitcher
Consultant Cardiologist, Worcestershire Royal Hospital, Worcester

Anthony D Redmond
Professor of Emergency Medicine, Keele University, and Consultant in Emergency Medicine, the North Staffordshire Hospital NHS Trust, Stoke on Trent

Sam Richmond
Consultant Neonatologist, Sunderland Royal Hospital, Sunderland

Robert Simons
Consultant Anaesthetist, Royal Free Hospital, London

Kenneth Spearpoint
Senior Resuscitation Officer, Hammersmith Hospitals NHS Trust, London

Mark Stacey
Consultant Obstetric Anaesthetist, Llandough Hospital and Community NHS Trust, South Glamorgan

Brian Steggles
Chairman, Faculty of Prehospital Care, Royal College of Surgeons, Edinburgh

Richard Vincent
Professor of Medicine, Brighton and Sussex Medical School, Brighton

A J Harry Walmsley
Clinical Director and Consultant in Anaesthetics, East Sussex Hospitals NHS Trust, Eastbourne

Jonathan Wylie
Consultant Neonatologist, The James Cook University Hospital, Middlesbrough

Geralyn Wynn
Resuscitation Training Officer, Royal Free Hospital, London

David A Zideman
Consultant Anaesthetist, Hammersmith Hospital NHS Trust, London

Introduction

The modern era of resuscitation began in 1960 with the publication of the classic paper by Jude, Kouwenhoven, and Knickerbocker on closed chest cardiac compression, which showed that the circulation could be maintained during cardiac arrest without the need for thoracotomy. A few years earlier Elam, Safar, and Gordon had established expired air ventilation as the most effective method for providing artificial ventilation for a patient who had stopped breathing. The effectiveness of closed chest defibrillation had been demonstrated by Zoll a few years earlier. By combining the techniques of chest compression with expired air ventilation, it became possible to maintain the viability of a patient in cardiopulmonary arrest until a defibrillator could be brought to the scene. Special units were established that were able to resuscitate patients at high risk of developing cardiac arrest, and special hospital cardiac arrest teams were created.

After coronary care units were established for patients with acute myocardial infarction, it became apparent that most deaths from the condition occurred in the early stages, not because the myocardium was severely damaged, but because of potentially treatable disturbances in the cardiac rhythm. Once the effectiveness of resuscitation in hospital was established, the realisation that two thirds of deaths from coronary heart disease occurred before hospital admission led to attempts to provide coronary care, and particularly defibrillation, in the community. The credit for this development goes to Pantridge in Belfast, who pioneered the first mobile coronary care unit staffed by a doctor and nurse. This early experience confirmed the high incidence of lethal arrhythmias at the onset of myocardial infarction and many patients attended by the mobile units were successfully resuscitated from cardiac arrest. Pantridge and his coworkers also drew attention to the value of cardiopulmonary resuscitation (CPR) performed by bystanders before the arrival of the mobile unit.

In the early 1970s, Leonard Cobb, a cardiologist in Seattle, inspired by these results, equipped paramedics with defibrillators and trained firefighters to act as first responders and perform basic life support. The fire service in Seattle is highly coordinated and a standard fire appliance can reach any part of the city within four minutes. CPR was, therefore, already in progress when more highly trained ambulance paramedics arrived some minutes later.

Two factors were found to be crucial determinants of survival from cardiac arrest. The first was the presence of bystanders able to perform basic life support. The second was the speed with which defibrillation was performed. To reduce this time interval further, the firefighters in Seattle were equipped with defibrillators, a process facilitated by the development of the semi-automatic advisory models that require less training to use.

Vickery, the chief of the fire service in Seattle, made the important suggestion that CPR by members of the public should be the first stage in the provision of coronary care outside hospital. Together with Cobb, he inaugurated training in resuscitation techniques for the public to further increase the practice of CPR. The widespread provision of bystander CPR in the community, coupled with the provision of prompt defibrillation, has resulted in survival rates of up to 40% being reported from that area of the United States.

In the United Kingdom, progress in community resuscitation was slower to gain momentum, but progress has been rapid in recent years. Scotland became the first country in the world to equip every emergency ambulance with a defibrillator. These are now standard equipment throughout the United Kingdom, with survival rates of up to 50% reported when cardiac arrest is witnessed by an ambulance crew. Initiatives to train the public in CPR techniques have proved popular and have made an important contribution to improved survival rates.

More recently, resuscitation in the community has made a crucial advance with the introduction of "public access defibrillation"—a concept intended to further reduce the delay in defibrillation by placing defibrillators in busy public places for use by trained lay people before the arrival of the ambulance service. The rhythm recognition algorithms in modern automated defibrillators have proved sufficiently accurate and the machines are simple to operate by suitably trained lay people. Some public access defibrillation programmes have reported impressive results and England now has the first national public access defibrillation programme in the world. The British Heart Foundation has been instrumental in supplying defibrillators for use by the public, and although public access defibrillation is in its early stages in the United Kingdom, several people who have collapsed at railway stations or airports have been resuscitated by lay people before the arrival of the emergency medical services.

Major efforts have been made to improve hospital resuscitation in the United Kingdom. Increasingly, proficiency in resuscitation skills is expected at postgraduate examinations and has been become a pre-requisite for appointment to many specialist posts. The automated defibrillator has enabled a wider range of staff to administer the first crucial shocks with the minimum of delay. In the ideal situation, a patient is promptly defibrillated by those present at the time of the arrest well before the arrival of the hospital cardiac arrest team. These may be junior medical or nursing staff with relatively limited experience.

The recognition that many hospital patients who suffer cardiopulmonary arrest display warning signs indicating an underlying deterioration in their clinical condition has led to a redefinition of the roles of hospital cardiac arrest team. Increasingly, medical emergency teams are called at the first appearance of such premonitory signs to prevent cardiac arrest by the intensive management of the factors complicating the patient's underlying condition. Should cardiac arrest occur the chances of resuscitation are increased by concentrating the experienced staff and equipment at the patient's bedside.

Training in resuscitation techniques for hospital staff has improved greatly with the appointment of specialist resuscitation training officers and the provision of standardised, validated, advanced life support courses available nationally. Separate courses administered by the Resuscitation Council (UK) teach adult, paediatric, or neonatal resuscitation.

The Resuscitation Council (UK) comprises doctors from many disciplines and others who share the desire to improve standards of resuscitation both in hospital and in the community. Members of the Resuscitation Council (UK), with invited experts, produced the first edition of the *ABC of Resuscitation* in 1986 with the intention that it should serve as a practical guide to resuscitation for the 1980s. The second, third, and fourth editions moved into the 1990s and it is our intention that the fifth edition will perform the same function in the new millennium.

Michael Colquhoun,
Chairman

Anthony J Handley
Chairman BLS and AED Subcommittee
Past Chairman

T R Evans
Past Chairman

Resuscitation Council (UK)
5th Floor
Tavistock House North
Tavistock Square
London WC1H 9HR

Telephone: 020 7388 4678,
Email: enquiries@resus.org.uk
Website: www.resus.org.uk

Introduction to the Fifth Edition

The formation of the International Liaison Committee on Resuscitation (ILCOR) in 1992 was a landmark in international cooperation to improve the management of patients who suffer cardiopulmonary arrest. By the second half of the 1990s, common resuscitation guidelines were in use throughout most of Europe and in many other countries worldwide. At the same time, it became widely recognised that there was inadequate scientific evidence on which to base recommendations for best practice in many areas of resuscitation.

During the late 1990s an extensive review was undertaken of the scientific evidence on which current resuscitation practice was based. Two international conferences, and extensive work by subcommittees that examined individual topics in detail, led to the publication of the *International Guidelines 2000*. This represents a consensus based on a critical evaluation of the scientific evidence on which current practice is based. New procedures had to pass a rigorous evidence-based evaluation before being recommended. Revision or deletion of some practices or procedures from the existing guidelines resulted when a lack of evidence confirmed the effectiveness of a procedure or when new evidence suggested harm or ineffectiveness, or indicated that superior therapies were now available. These guidelines are seen as the most effective and easily teachable resuscitation guidelines that current knowledge, research, and experience can provide.

In the fifth edition of the *ABC of Resuscitation*, the guidelines and treatment algorithms recommended are based on guidelines published by the European Resuscitation Council and the Resuscitation Council (UK), which are, in turn, derived from the *International Guidelines 2000 Consensus on Science*.

Reference

International Guidelines 2000 for cardiopulmonary resuscitation and emergency cardiovascular care—an international consensus on science. *Resuscitation* 2000;46:1-448
Resuscitation Guidelines 2000. London: Resuscitation Council (UK), 2000.

Michael Colquhoun
Chairman of the Resuscitation Council (UK) and Chairman,
Research Subcommittee

Anthony J Handley
Past Chairman, Resuscitation Council (UK) and Chairman of ILCOR
Working Party on Basic Life Support

T R Evans
Past Chairman, Resuscitation Council (UK)

Notes on the algorithm approach to resuscitation

Resuscitation algorithms first appeared during the 1980s and have become a major method used to depict critical points in the assessment and treatment of victims of cardiac arrest. They serve as educational tools and are designed to act as *aides mémoires* to assist the performance of rescuers, providing a convenient and illustrative summary of large amounts of information. They are not designed, however, to be comprehensive or proscriptive; the clinician in charge should always determine whether a step in an algorithm is appropriate for an individual patient, and should be prepared to deviate from the algorithm if the patient's condition requires this. It is not expected that all the algorithms will be memorised in all their detail. They provide a ready source of reference to lead the clinician through the process of assessment and treatment necessary during a resuscitation procedure.

The following important recommendations apply to the interpretation of all resuscitation algorithms:

- Treat the patient not the monitor
- When proceeding through an algorithm it is assumed that the previous stage has been unsuccessful, and that the patient remains in cardiac arrest
- The algorithms assume that basic life support is always performed
- Interventions should only be undertaken when an appropriate indication exists
- Most of the stages in the algorithms are based on procedures for which there is good scientific evidence of effectiveness. Procedures that are less likely to be effective but which are worthy of consideration are contained in footnotes
- The provision of an adequate airway, ventilation, and oxygenation with chest compression and defibrillation are considered the more important interventions and take precedence over establishing intravenous access or the administration of drugs
- Several drugs, such as adrenaline (epinephrine), lignocaine (lidocaine) and atropine can be administered via the tracheal tube when intravenous access is not available. The endotracheal dose is 2-2.5 × the intravenous dose and should be diluted in an adequate quantity (10 ml) of carrier fluid
- Where a peripheral intravenous line is employed, intravenous drugs should usually be administered rapidly as a bolus and followed with a 20-30 ml bolus of intravenous fluid to enhance delivery into the central circulation

Acknowledgements

The editors are grateful to the following companies for their help with illustrations of equipment.

Ambu Ltd, St Ives, Cambridgeshire; Medtronic Physio Control, Watford; Cook Critical Care (UK), Letchford, Hertfordshire; Laerdal Medical Ltd, Orpington, Kent; Medtronic, Watford, Hertfordshire; St Jude, Coventry, Warickshire; Vitalograph Ltd, Maids Moreton, Buckingham; Zoll Medical (UK) Ltd, Manchester. The figure of implantable cardioverter defibrillators from 1992 and 2002 is supplied by C D Finlay, CRT coordinator, Guidant Canada Corporation, Toronto.

The diagram of a laryngeal mask airway in situ on page 30 is adapted from Kirk RM, ed. *General surgical operations*. London: Churchill Livingstone, 1987.

We would like to thank the following people for their help in providing photographs: Michael Colquhoun; Cliff Randall, Welsh Ambulance Service NHS Trust; Dr Rupert Evans and staff of the accident and emergency department, University Hospital of Wales, Cardiff; the resuscitation training department, Worcester Royal Hospitals, Worcester; Gavin D Perkins, Simon Giles, and John Dodds at Birmingham Heartlands Hospital.

Thanks also to Judy Wood and Linda Sullivan for their secretarial help.

1   Basic life support

Anthony J Handley

Basic life support is the maintenance of an airway and the support of breathing and the circulation without using equipment other than a simple airway device or protective shield. A combination of expired air ventilation (rescue breathing) and chest compression is known as cardiopulmonary resuscitation (CPR), which forms the basis of modern basic life support. The term "cardiac arrest" implies a sudden interruption of cardiac output, which may be reversible with appropriate treatment. It does not include the cessation of heart activity as a terminal event in serious illness; in these circumstances the techniques of basic life support are usually inappropriate.

Survival after cardiac arrest is most likely to be the outcome in the following circumstances: when the event is witnessed; when a bystander summons help from the emergency services and starts resuscitation; when the heart arrests in ventricular fibrillation; and when defibrillation and advanced life support are instituted at an early stage. Basic life support is one link in this chain of survival. It entails assessment followed by action—the ABC: A is for assessment and airway, B is for breathing, and C is for circulation.

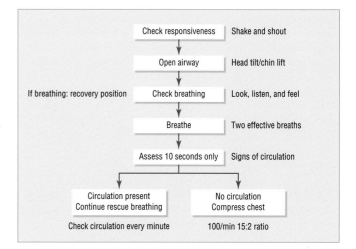

Adult basic life support. Send or go for help as soon as possible according to guidelines. Adapted from *Resuscitation Guidelines 2000*, London: Resuscitation Council (UK), 2000

Assessment

Rapidly assess any danger to the patient and yourself from hazards such as falling masonry, gas, electricity, fire, or traffic because there is no sense in having two patients. Establish whether the patient is responsive by gently shaking his or her shoulders and asking loudly "Are you all right?" Be careful not to aggravate any existing injury, particularly of the cervical spine.

If no response is given, shout for help

Airway

Establishing and maintaining an airway is the single most useful manoeuvre that the rescuer can perform.

Loosen tight clothing around the patient's neck. Extend, but do not hyperextend, the neck, thus lifting the tongue off the posterior wall of the pharynx. This is best achieved by placing your hand on the patient's upper forehead and exerting pressure to tilt the head. Remove any obvious obstruction from the mouth; leave well fitting dentures in place. Place two fingertips under the point of the chin to lift it forwards. This will often allow breathing to restart.

Look, listen, and feel for breathing: look for chest movement, listen close to the mouth for breath sounds, and feel for air with your cheek. Look, listen, and feel for 10 seconds before deciding that breathing is absent.

Recovery position
If the patient is unconscious but is breathing, place him or her in the recovery position. If necessary, support the chin to maintain an airway. In this position the tongue will fall away from the pharyngeal wall and any vomit or secretion will dribble out of the corner of the mouth rather than obstruct the airway or, later on, cause aspiration.

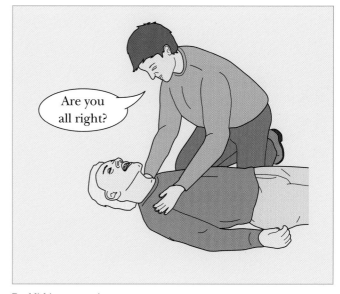

Establishing responsiveness

Breathing

If breathing is absent, send a bystander to telephone for an ambulance. If you are on your own, go yourself. The exception to this rule is when the patient is a child or the cause of the patient's collapse is near drowning, drug or alcohol intoxication, trauma, or choking. Under these circumstances it is likely that you are dealing with a primary respiratory arrest and appropriate resuscitation should be given for about one minute before seeking help.

Return to the patient and maintain an airway by tilting the head and lifting the chin. Pinch the nose closed with the fingers of your hand on the forehead. Take a breath, seal your lips firmly around those of the patient, and breathe out until you see the patient's chest clearly rising. It is important for each full breath to last about two seconds. Lift your head away, watching the patient's chest fall, and take another breath of air. The chest should rise as you blow in and fall when you take your mouth away. Each breath should expand the patient's chest visibly but not cause overinflation as this will allow air to enter the oesophagus and stomach. Subsequent gastric distension causes not only vomiting but also passive regurgitation into the lungs, which often goes undetected.

If the patient is still not breathing after two rescue breaths (or after five attempts at ventilation, even if unsuccessful), check for signs of a circulation. Look and listen for any movement, breathing (other than an occasional gasp), or coughing. Take no more than 10 seconds to make your check.

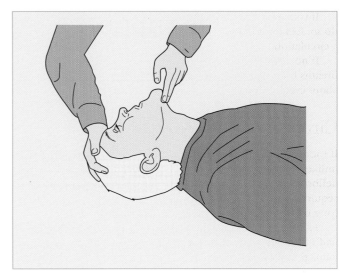

Head tilt and jaw lift

The best pulse to feel in an emergency is the carotid pulse, but if the neck is injured the femoral pulse may be felt at the groin

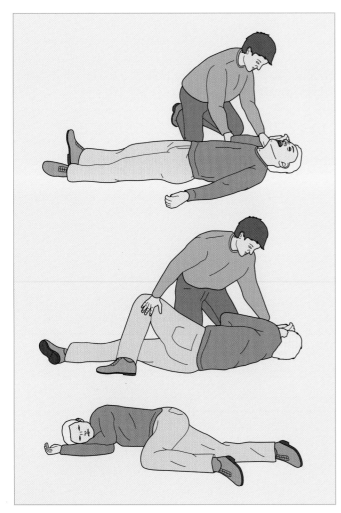

Turning casualty into the recovery position

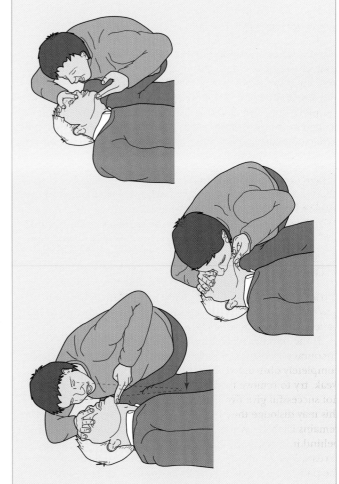

Expired air resuscitation

If you are a healthcare provider, and have been trained to do so, feel for a pulse as part of your check for signs of a circulation.

If no signs of a circulation are present continue with rescue breaths but recheck the circulation after every 10 breaths or about every minute.

Circulation

If there are no signs of a circulation (cardiac arrest) it is unlikely that the patient will recover as a result of CPR alone, so defibrillation and other advanced life support are urgently required. Ensure that the patient is on his or her back and lying on a firm, flat surface, then start chest compressions.

The correct place to compress is in the centre of the lower half of the sternum. To find this, and to ensure that the risk of damaging intra-abdominal organs is minimised, feel along the rib margin until you come to the xiphisternum. Place your middle finger on the xiphisternum and your index finger on the bony sternum above, then slide the heel of your other hand down to these fingers and leave it there. Remove your first hand and place it on top of the second. Press down firmly, keeping your arms straight and elbows locked. In an adult compress about 4-5 cm, keeping the pressure firm, controlled, and applied vertically. Try to spend about the same amount of time in the compressed phase as in the released phase and aim for a rate of 100 compressions/min (a little less than two compressions per second). After every 15 compressions tilt the head, lift the chin, and give two rescue breaths. Return your hands immediately to the sternum and give 15 further compressions, continuing compressions and rescue breaths in a ratio of 15:2. It may help to get the right rate and ratio by counting: "One, two, three, four ...."

If two trained rescuers are present one should assume responsibility for rescue breaths and the other for chest compression. The compression rate should remain at 100/min, but there should be a pause after every 15 compressions that is just long enough to allow two rescue breaths to be given, lasting two seconds each. Provided the patient's airway is maintained it is not necessary to wait for exhalation before resuming chest compressions.

Precordial thump

Studies have shown that an initial precordial (chest) thump may restart the recently arrested heart. This is particularly the case if the onset of cardiac arrest is witnessed.

Choking

A patient who is choking may have been seen eating or a child may have put an object into his or her mouth. Often the patient grips his or her throat with their hand.

If the patient is still breathing, he or she should be encouraged to continue coughing. If the flow of air is completely obstructed, or the patient shows signs of becoming weak, try to remove the foreign body from the mouth. If this is not successful give five firm back blows between the scapulae; this may dislodge the obstruction by compressing the air that remains in the lungs, thereby producing an upward force behind it. If this fails to clear the airway then try five abdominal thrusts. Make a fist of one of your hands and place it just below the patient's xiphisternum. Grasp this fist with your other hand and push firmly and suddenly upwards and posteriorly. Then alternate abdominal thrusts with back slaps.

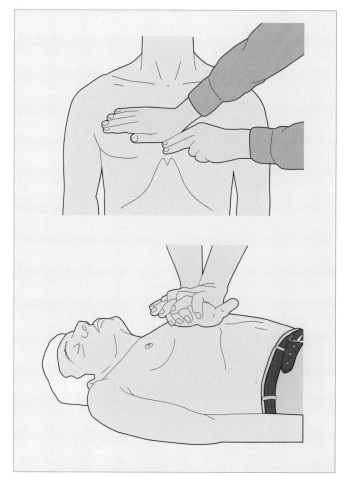

Hand position for chest compression

The precordial thump is taught as a standard part of advanced life support

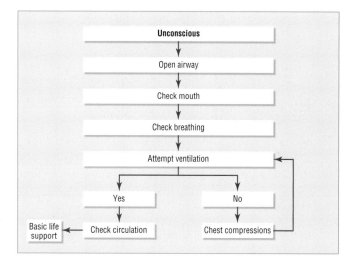

Management of choking in adults. Adapted from *Resuscitation Guidelines 2000*, London: Resuscitation Council (UK), 2000

If a choking patient becomes unconscious, this may result in the muscles around the larynx relaxing enough to allow air past the obstruction. If breathing does not resume, open the patient's airway by lifting the chin and tilting the head, and then attempt to give two effective rescue breaths. If this fails, start chest compressions, alternating 15 compressions with a further attempt to give rescue breaths. In this situation, the chest compressions are given to relieve airway obstruction rather than to circulate the blood as in cardiac arrest.

Dangers of resuscitation

Until fairly recently the main concern in resuscitation was for the patient, but attention has now been directed towards the rescuer, particularly in the light of fears about the transmission of AIDS. However, no case of AIDS due to transfer from patient to rescuer (or vice versa) by mouth to mouth resuscitation has been reported. Despite the presence of the virus in saliva, it does not seem that transmission occurs via this route in the absence of blood to blood contact. Nevertheless, there is still concern about the possible risk of infection, and those who may be called on to administer resuscitation should be allowed to use some form of barrier device. This may take the form of a ventilation mask (for mouth to mask ventilation) or a filter device placed over the mouth and nose. The main requirement of these devices is that they should not hinder an adequate flow of air and not provide too large a dead space. Resuscitation must not be delayed while such a device is being sought.

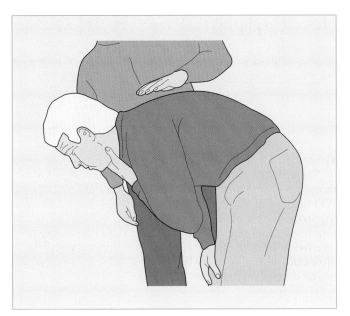

Choking and back blows

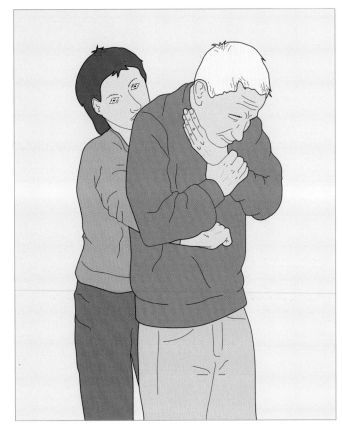

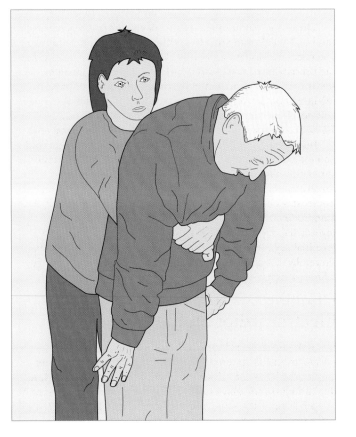

Abdominal thrusts in a conscious patient

Further reading

- Handley AJ, Monsieurs KG, Bossaert LL. European Resuscitation Council guidelines 2000 for adult basic life support. *Resuscitation* 2001;48:199-205.
- Ornato JP. Efficacy vs. effectiveness: The case of active compression-decompression (ACD) CPR. *Resuscitation* 1997;34:3-4.
- International guidelines 2000 for cardiopulmonary resuscitation and emergency cardiovascular care—an international consensus on science. Part 3: adult basic life support. *Resuscitation* 2000; 46:29-71.

2 Ventricular fibrillation

Michael Colquhoun, Charles D Deakin, Douglas Chamberlain

The normal cardiac cycle is controlled by an orderly sequence of depolarisation spreading into the ventricular myocardium through specialised conducting tissue. In ventricular fibrillation (VF) this coordinated sequence is lost and individual muscle cells depolarise in an apparently random fashion with the loss of all coordinated muscular activity. The heart stops functioning as an effective pump and, in the absence of cardiac output, the myocardium becomes more ischaemic and irreversible cerebral anoxic damage occurs within a few minutes.

> **The definite treatment for VF is to apply an electrical countershock from a defibrillator**

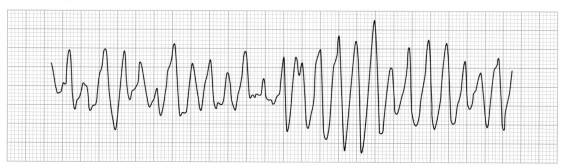

Onset

The sooner an electrical countershock from a defibrillator can be given after the onset of VF, then the greater the chance of successful defibrillation. Several clinical studies have shown that the probability of successful defibrillation and subsequent survival to hospital discharge is inversely related to the time interval between the onset of VF and delivery of the first countershock. The chance of success declines by about 7-10% for each minute delay in administering the shock.

During VF the myocardial cells continue to contract rapidly and exhaust the limited oxygen and high energy phosphate stores contained in the cells, which are not replenished. Anaerobic metabolism results in intracellular acidosis as cellular homeostasis breaks down. In the absence of defibrillation, the amplitude of the fibrillatory waveform decreases progressively as myocardial oxygen and energy reserves are exhausted and terminal asystole eventually supervenes. This process may be slowed by effective basic life support techniques that provide a limited supply of blood to the myocardium.

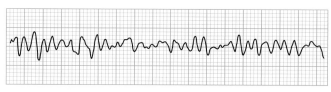

Five minutes

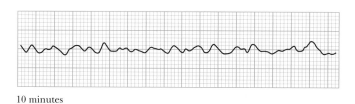

10 minutes

Electrocardiographic appearances

In VF the electrocardiograph shows a bizarre, irregular waveform that is apparently random in both frequency and amplitude. VF is sometimes classified as either coarse or fine, depending on the amplitude of the complexes. The treatment of each form is the same and the only practical implication of a distinction is to give some indication of the potential for successful defibrillation and to serve as a reminder that VF may be mistaken for asystole.

Epidemiology

VF is the commonest initial rhythm leading to cardiac arrest, particularly in patients with coronary heart disease. VF may be

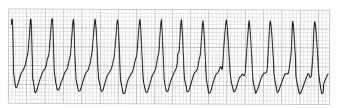

Pulseless ventricular tachycardia is treated in the same way as VF

preceded by ventricular tachycardia and is seen in up to
80-90% of those patients dying suddenly outside hospital in
whom the cardiac rhythm can be monitored without delay. It is
particularly common in the early stages of myocardial
infarction. It is therefore important that those general
practitioners and ambulance staff who are often the first to
attend to such patients should carry defibrillators. Considerable
effort is being devoted to training members of the public to
carry out basic life support to extend the window of
opportunity for successful defibrillation. This has been effective
in reducing the delay in defibrillation, and impressive rates of
successful resuscitation have been reported.

Electrical defibrillation

Electrical defibrillation is the only reliable method of
defibrillation; no drug has a consistent defibrillatory effect.
Defibrillation aims to depolarise most of the myocardium
simultaneously, thereby allowing the natural pacemaker tissue
to resume control of the heart. Depolarisation of a critical mass
of myocardium is necessary and this depends on the
transmyocardial current flow (measured in Amperes) rather
than the energy of the delivered shock (measured in Joules).

A precordial thump may occasionally abolish ventricular
tachycardia or VF by generating a small intrinsic electrical
current within the heart. This technique is most likely to be
successful if applied very soon after onset of the arrythmia, so a
thump should be considered in cases of witnessed, particularly
monitored, cardiac arrest.

History of defibrillation

Prevost and Batelli are usually credited with the discovery in
1900 that VF could be reversed by defibrillation. They were able
to initiate and abolish fibrillation in experimental animals by the
application of AC and DC shocks. Their work remained
dormant for many years, probably because the importance of
VF in humans was not recognised until the 1940s. Wiggers
repeated their work in the 1930s, which then prompted Claude
Beck, a surgeon in Cleveland, to attempt defibrillation in
humans who developed VF while undergoing thoracotomy.
Between 1937 and 1947 Beck made several unsuccessful
attempts using a homemade AC defibrillator, developed by
Kouwenhoven, with electrodes placed directly on the heart.
His first success came in 1947 when VF developed in a 14 year
old boy whose chest was being closed after surgery for funnel
chest. Kouwenhoven was also instrumental in the development
of the external defibrillator, which was first successfully
employed by Paul Zoll in a patient with recurrent VF and
pulseless ventricular tachycardia complicating sinoatrial disease.
The first successful defibrillation outside hospital was reported
by Pantridge in 1967

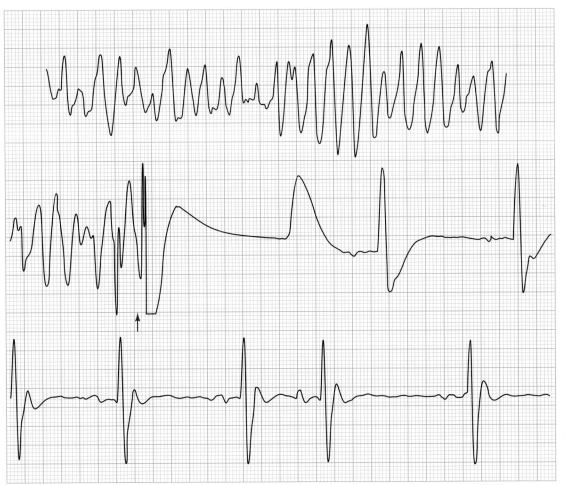

A continuous
electrocardiogram
recording showing the
successful treatment of
VF by a countershock
(delivered at the arrow)

Factors influencing defibrillation

Transmyocardial current flow

A shock that is too low in energy may result in a current flow that is inadequate to achieve successful defibrillation. Higher energy shocks may result in greater current flow but carry the risk of causing damage if the current is too high. The optimal shock energy is one that will achieve defibrillation successfully while causing minimal electrical injury to the myocardium. Achieving an appropriate current flow will reduce the number of shocks required and may limit further myocardial damage.

The magnitude of the current passing through the heart will depend on the voltage delivered by the defibrillator and the transthoracic impedance—that is, the resistance to current flow through the chest wall, lungs, and myocardium. The relationship between these factors can be expressed by a simple mathematical equation.

Transthoracic impedence

In adults transthoracic impedence averages about 60 Ohms, with 95% of the population lying in the range of 30-90 Ohms.

Current flow will be highest when transthoracic impedence is at its lowest. To achieve this the operator should press firmly when using handheld electrode paddles. A conductive electrode gel or defibrillator pads should be used to reduce the impedance at the electrode and skin interface. Self-adhesive monitor or defibrillator electrodes do not require additional pressure. In patients with considerable chest hair, poor electrode contact and air trapping will increase the impedance. This can be avoided by rapidly shaving the chest in the areas where the electrodes are placed. Transthoracic impedance is about 9% lower when the lungs are empty, so defibrillation is best carried out during the expiratory phase of ventilation. It is also important to avoid positioning the electrodes over the breast tissue of female patients because this causes high impedance to current flow.

Defibrillator shock waveform

The effectiveness of a shock in terminating VF depends on the type of shock waveform discharged by the defibrillator. Traditionally, defibrillators delivered a monophasic sinusoidal or damped sinusoidal waveform. Recently it has been shown that biphasic waveforms (in which the polarity of the shock changes) are more effective than monophasic shocks of equivalent energy. Defibrillators that deliver biphasic shocks are now in clinical use, and considerable savings in size and weight result from the reduced energy levels needed. Biphasic shocks have been widely employed in implantable cardioverter defibrillators (ICDs) because their increased effectiveness allows more shocks to be given for any particular battery size.

Defibrillators that use biphasic waveforms offer the potential of both greater efficiency and less myocardial damage than conventional monophasic defibrillators. Much of this evidence has been gained from studies conducted during the implantation of cardioverter defibrillators but some evidence shows that the increased efficiency of biphasic waveforms leads to higher survival rates during resuscitation attempts.

Energy levels

The likelihood of successful defibrillation depends, to some extent, on chance. For example, a success rate of 70% means failure in 30 out of 100 patients. If a further shock, with the same 70% chance of success, is given to those 30 patients an additional 21 successes will be achieved (70% of 30).

When using a defibrillator with a monomorphic waveform it is recommended that the first shock should be at an energy

---

Determinants of current flow

- Energy of delivered shock
- Transthoracic impedance
- Electrode position
- Shock waveform
- Body size
- Electrode size

Determinants of current flow

$$I \propto \frac{\sqrt{E}}{TTI}$$

I = peak discharge current
E = energy selected
TTI = transthoracic impedance

Determinants of transthoracic impedence

- Shock energy
- Electrode size
- Electrical contact
- Number of and time since previous shocks
- Phase of ventilation
- Distance between electrodes
- Paddle or electrode pressure

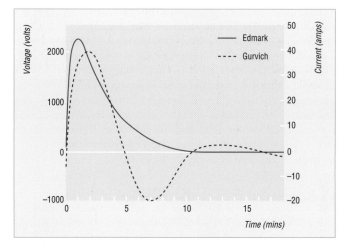

Edmark monophasic and Gurvich biphasic defibrillator waveforms

level of 200 J. Should this be unsuccessful, a second shock at the same energy level may prove effective because the transthoracic impedance is reduced by repeated shocks. If two shocks at 200 J are unsuccessful, the energy setting should be increased to 360 J for the third and subsequent attempts.

Current guidelines recommend that biphasic shocks of equivalent effectiveness to monophasic shocks may be used during resuscitation attempts. Although this equivalence is not clearly defined, and may vary between different types of biphasic waveform, a biphasic shock of 150 J is commonly considered to be at least as effective as a 200 J monophasic shock. Many automated biphasic defibrillators do not employ escalating shock energies and have produced similar clinical outcomes to the use of conventional monophasic defibrillators in which the third and subsequent shocks are delivered at 360 J.

Technological advances

The most important technological advance in recent times has been the introduction of defibrillators that incorporate biphasic waveform technology. Another technique to increase efficiency is the use of sequentially overlapping shocks that produce a shifting electrical vector during a multiple pulse shock. This technique may also reduce the energy requirements for successful defibrillation.

Defibrillators have also been developed that measure the transthoracic impedance and then deliver a current determined by this. The optimal current for terminating VF lies between 30 and 40 Amperes with a monophasic damped sinusoidal waveform. Studies are in progress to determine the equivalent current dosages for biphasic shocks.

Manual defibrillation

Manual defibrillators use electrical energy from batteries or from the mains to charge a capacitor, and the energy stored is then subsequently discharged through electrodes placed on the casualty's chest. These may either be handheld paddles or electrodes similar to the adhesive electrodes used with automated defibrillators. The energy stored in the capacitor may be varied by a manual control on which the calibration points indicate the energy in Joules delivered by the machine.

Modern defibrillators allow monitoring of the electrocardiogram (ECG) through the defibrillator electrodes and display the rhythm on a screen. With a manual defibrillator, the operator interprets the rhythm and decides if a shock is required. The strength of the shock, the charging of the capacitor, and the delivery of the shock are all under the control of the operator. Most modern machines allow these procedures to be performed through controls contained in the handles of the paddles so that the procedure may be accomplished without removing the electrodes from the chest wall. Considerable skill and training are required, mainly because of the need to interpret the ECG.

Procedure for defibrillation

The universal algorithm for the management of cardiac arrest is designed to be used with both manual and automated defibrillators. In this chapter we cover the procedures recommended for manual defibrillation. The use of automated defibrillators is covered in Chapter 3.

Recognising the importance of reducing to a minimum the delay between onset of VF and the application of a defibrillatory shock, the patient's rhythm should be determined

Electrode position
- The ideal electrode position allows maximum current to flow through the myocardium. This will occur when the heart lies in the direct path of the current
- The standard position consists of one electrode placed to the right of the upper sternum below the right clavicle and the other placed in the midaxillary line at the level of the fifth left intercostal space
- An alternative is to place one electrode to the left of the lower sternal border and the other on the posterior chest wall below the angle of the left scapula
- Avoid placing electrodes directly over breast tissue in women

Electrode size or surface area
- Low transthoracic impedence is achieved with larger electrodes
- Above an optimum size the transmyocardial current will be reduced
- The usual electrode sizes employed are 10-13 cm in diameter for adults and 4.5-8 cm for infants and children

Body size
- Infants and children require shocks of lower energy than adults to achieve defibrillation
- Over the usual range of weight encountered in adults, body size does not greatly influence the energy requirements

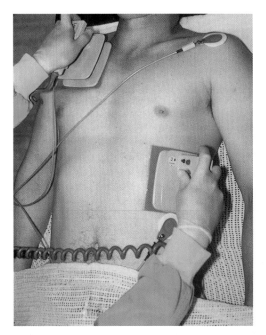

Manual defibrillation

With a manual defibrillator, the cardiac rhythm may be monitored through the paddles or adhesive electrodes placed on the chest in the position where a shock will then be given

at the earliest possible opportunity. Basic life support should be started if the defibrillator is not available immediately, but it should not delay delivery of the shock. If the arrest was witnessed, particularly in patients who are already monitored, and a defibrillator is not immediately available, a precordial thump should be given.

In the presence of VF (or pulseless ventricular tachycardia) the left-hand side of the universal algorithm should be followed. Up to three shocks are given initially. In machines that deliver a monophasic waveform, energy levels of 200 J, 200 J, and 360 J should be used. Shocks of equivalent energy should be used with defibrillators that administer biphasic shocks. If more than one shock is required, the paddles or adhesive electrodes should be left in position on the patient's chest while the defibrillator is recharged, and the monitor observed for any change in rhythm. When all three shocks are required, the objective should be to deliver these within one minute. This sequence should not normally need to be interrupted by basic life support, but if a delay occurs, because the equipment available does not permit rapid recharging between shocks, it is appropriate to consider providing basic life support between shocks.

The carotid pulse should be checked only if the ECG changes to a rhythm compatible with a cardiac output. However, it is important to remember that after a shock is given a delay of a few seconds often occurs before the ECG display is again of diagnostic quality. In addition, successful defibrillation is often followed by a period of apparent asystole before a coordinated rhythm is established. Even if a rhythm that is normally compatible with a cardiac output is obtained, a period of impaired myocardial contractility often occurs, resulting in a weak or impalpable carotid pulse. It is important not to make a spurious diagnosis of pulseless electrical activity under these circumstances; for this reason the algorithm recommends only one minute of cardiopulmonary resuscitation (CPR) before reassessment of the rhythm and a further pulse check.

After tracheal intubation chest compressions should continue uninterrupted at a rate of 100 per minute (except for defibrillation, pulse checks, or other procedures), while ventilation is continued at a rate of about 12 ventilations per minute. Continuous chest compressions may be possible with a laryngeal mask airway (LMA), but the seal around the larynx must prevent gas leaking and permit adequate ventilation of the lungs. If this is not possible, chest compressions should be interrupted to allow the usual 15:2 compression:ventilation ratio.

Intravenous access should be established at an early stage in the management of cardiac arrest. Although cannulation of the central veins allows drugs to be delivered rapidly into the circulation, more complications can occur, some of which are serious. In most circumstances peripheral venous cannulation is quicker, easier, and safer. The choice will be determined by the skills of those present and the equipment available.

In recent recommendations on the treatment of patients with VF refractory to initial attempts at defibrillation, anti-arrhythmic drugs have achieved less prominence. Amiodarone is currently recommended in the United Kingdom as the agent most likely to be successful in this situation. Lidocaine (lignocaine) may be considered as an alternative if amiodarone is not available but should not be given if the patient has previously received amiodarone. Procainamide is another alternative, although it is not widely employed in the United Kingdom. Further information about vasoconstrictor drugs and anti-arrhythmic agents is given in Chapter 16.

If the patient remains in VF after one minute of CPR, then up to three further shocks should be given, each at 360 J (or the equivalent with a biphasic defibrillator), and the

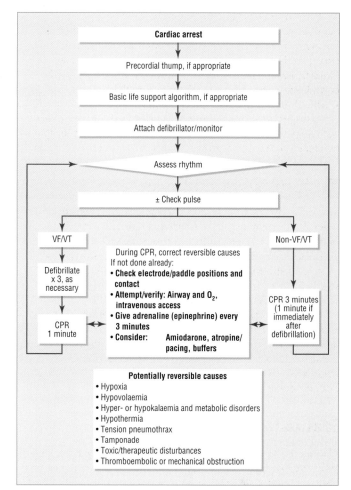

The advanced life support algorithm for the management of cardiac arrest in adults. Adapted from *Resuscitation Guidelines 2000*, London: Resuscitation Council (UK), 2000

The patient's airway should be secured. Tracheal intubation is the preferred method, but this depends on the experience of the rescuer; the LMA or Combi-tube are acceptable alternatives. Once the airway is secure, ventilation is performed with as high a concentration of oxygen as possible

With each loop of the algorithm 1 mg of adrenaline (epinephrine) should be administered. Vasopressin in a single intravenous dose of 40 units has recently been proposed as an alternative pending the outcome of further assessment of its role

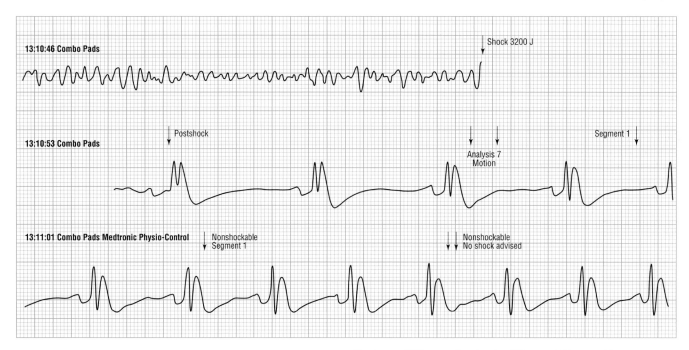

13:10:46 Combo Pads

Shock 3200 J

13:10:53 Combo Pads

Postshock

Analysis 7
Motion

Segment 1

13:11:01 Combo Pads Medtronic Physio-Control

Nonshockable
Segment 1

Nonshockable
No shock advised

Continuous ECG recording showing VF successfully treated by a countershock

monitor must be checked between each shock. The interval between batches of shocks should not exceed one minute, even if the airway has not been secured or intravenous access obtained, because the best chance of successful resuscitation still rests with defibrillation.

The loop on the left-hand side of the algorithm is continued with each sequence of three shocks (assuming successful defibrillation does not occur), which is followed by one minute of CPR. Further attempts to secure the airway or gain intravenous access may be attempted if necessary. Adrenaline (epinephrine) should be given with each loop or about every three minutes.

The use of alkalising or buffering agents has achieved less prominence in resuscitation guidelines in recent years. The use of bicarbonate may be considered if the arterial pH is less than 7.1 (or $[H]^+ > 0.80 \, mol/l$), if cardiac arrest is associated with overdose of tricyclic drugs or in the presence of hyperkalaemia. An initial dose of 50 mmol is used, with further doses determined by the results of blood gas analysis.

If VF persists, the position of the paddles may be changed or a different defibrillator, or paddles, or both, may be tried. Drugs given intravenously may take several minutes to exert their full effect, and drugs given by the endobronchial route may take even longer. Nothing is gained, however, by delaying further shocks because defibrillation remains the only intervention capable of restoring a spontaneous circulation. The algorithms are not intended to preclude the use of agents such as calcium, magnesium, or potassium salts whether for the treatment of known deficiencies in a particular patient, on clinical suspicion (for example, magnesium deficiency in patients on long-term diuretics), or on an empirical basis.

Safety

Care is needed to ensure that use of the defibrillator does not pose a risk to any of the staff participating in the resuscitation attempt. When defibrillation is carried out, it is essential that no part of any member of the team is in direct contact with the patient. The operator must shout "stand clear" and check that all those present have done so before giving the shock. There are traps for the unwary: wet surroundings or clothing are dangerous; intravenous infusion equipment must not be held

Defibrillation—points to note

- The number of "loops" completed during any particular cardiac arrest is a matter of judgment based on the clinical state of the patient and the prospects for a successful outcome
- Resuscitation that was started appropriately should not be abandoned while the rhythm is still recognisable VF; the development of persistent asystole is an indication that the prospects of success are poor
- Few situations call for resuscitation efforts continuing for more than one hour, exceptions being cardiac arrest in children, after drowning, or in the presence of hypothermia or drug overdose

Epidemiology of ventricular fibrillation

- 70 000 deaths per annum in the United Kingdom are sudden cardiac deaths
- Most sudden deaths are due to coronary disease
- Most coronary deaths occur outside hospital
- 50% of those who die of acute myocardial infarction do so within an hour of the onset
- VF rhythm at onset in 85-90% of patients

by assistants; the operator must be certain not to touch any part of the electrode surface; care is needed to ensure that excess electrode gel does not allow an electrical arc to form across the surface of the chest wall; and care is needed to ensure that the electrode gel does not spread from the chest wall to the operator's hands.

The use of gel defibrillator pads reduces the last two risks considerably. If the patient has a glyceryl trinitrate patch fitted then this should be removed before attempting defibrillation because an apparent explosion may occur if current is conducted through the foil backing used in some preparations.

Further reading

- Cummins RO, Hazinski MF, Kerber RE, Kudenchuk P, Becker L, Nichol G, et al. Low-energy biphasic waveform defibrillation: evidence based review. *Circulation* 1998;97:1654-67.
- Cummins RO, Ornato JP, Thies WH, Pepe PE. Improving survival from sudden cardiac arrest: the "chain of survival" concept: a statement for health professionals from the Advanced Life Support Subcommittee and the Emergency Cardiac Care Committee of the American Heart Association. *Circulation* 1991;83:1832-47.
- De Latorre F, Nolan J, Robertson C, Chamberlain D, Baskett P. European Resuscitation Council Guidelines 2000 for adult advanced life support. *Resuscitation* 2001;48:211-21.
- Eisenberg MS, Copass MK, Hallstrom AP, Blake B, Bergner L, Short FA, et al. Treatment of out-of-hospital cardiac arrest by rapid defibrillation by emergency medical technicians. *N Engl J Med* 1980;302:1379-83.
- International guidelines 2000 for cardiopulmonary resuscitation and emergency cardiac care—an international consensus on science. *Resuscitation* 2000;46:109-13 (Defibrillation), 167-8 (The algorithm approach to ACLS emergencies), 169-84 (A guide to the international ACLS algorithms).
- Pantridge JF, Geddes JS. A mobile intensive care unit in the management of myocardial infarction. *Lancet* 1967;II:271.
- Robertson C, Pre-cordial thump and cough techniques in advanced life support. *Resuscitation* 1992;24:133-5.
- Safar P. History of cardiopulmonary—cerebral resuscitation. In *Cardiopulmonary resuscitation*. Kaye W, Bircher NG, eds. London: Churchill Livingstone, 1989.
- Weaver WD, Cobb LA, Hallstrom AP, Farhrenbruch C, Copass MK, Factors influencing survival after out-of-hospital cardiac arrest. *J Am Coll Cardiol* 1986;7:752-7.
- Zoll P, Linenthal AJ, Gibson W, Paul MH, Normal LR. Termination of ventricular fibrillation in man by externally applied countershock. *N Engl J Med* 1956;254:727-32.

3 The automated external defibrillator

Roy Liddle, C Sian Davies, Michael Colquhoun, Anthony J Handley

The principles of electrical defibrillation of the heart and the use of manual defibrillators have been covered in Chapter 2. In this chapter we describe the automated external defibrillator (AED), which is generally considered to be the most important development in defibrillator technology in recent years.

Development of the AED

AED development came about through the recognition that, in adults, the commonest primary arrhythmia at the onset of cardiac arrest is ventricular fibrillation (VF) or pulseless ventricular tachycardia (VT). Survival is crucially dependent on minimising the delay before providing definitive therapy with a countershock. Use of a manual defibrillator requires considerable training, particularly in the skills of electrocardiogram (ECG) interpretation, and this greatly restricts the availability of prompt electrical treatment for these life-threatening arrhythmias.

In many cases conventional emergency medical systems cannot respond rapidly enough to provide defibrillation within the accepted time frame of eight minutes or less. This has led to an investigation into ways of automating the process of defibrillation so that defibrillators might be used by more people and, therefore, be more widely deployed in the community.

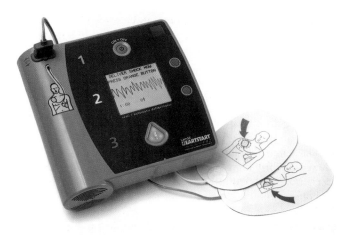

Modern AED

Principles of automated defibrillation

When using an AED many of the stages in performing defibrillation are automated. All that is required of the operator is to recognise that cardiac arrest may have occurred and to attach two adhesive electrodes to the patient's chest. These electrodes serve a dual function, allowing the ECG to be recorded and a shock to be given should it be indicated. The process of ECG interpretation is undertaken automatically and if the sophisticated electronic algorithm in the device detects VF (or certain types of VT) the machine charges itself automatically to a predetermined level. Some models also display the ECG rhythm on a monitor screen.

When fully charged, the device indicates to the operator that a shock should be given. Full instructions are provided by

The International 2000 guidelines for cardiopulmonary resuscitation (CPR) and emergency cardiac care recommend that healthcare workers with a duty to perform CPR should be trained, equipped, and authorised to perform defibrillation

Public access defibrillation should be established:
- When the frequency of cardiac arrest is such that there is a reasonable probability of the use of an AED within five years
- When a paramedic response time of less than five minutes cannot be achieved
- When the AED can be delivered to the patient within five minutes

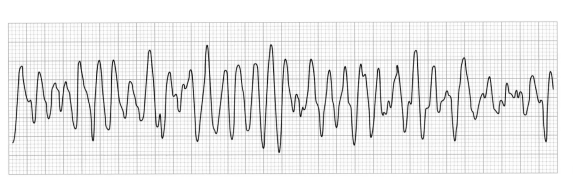

Ventricular fibrillation

voice prompts and written instructions on a screen. Some models feature a simple 1-2-3 numerical scheme to indicate the next procedure required, and most illuminate the control that administers the shock. After the shock has been delivered, the AED will analyse the ECG again and if VF persists the process is repeated up to a maximum of three times in any one cycle. AEDs are programmed to deliver shocks in groups of three in accordance with current guidelines. If the third shock is unsuccessful the machine will then indicate that CPR should be performed for a period (usually one minute) after which the device will instruct rescuers to stand clear while it reanalyses the rhythm. If the arrhythmia persists, the machine will charge itself and indicate that a further shock is required.

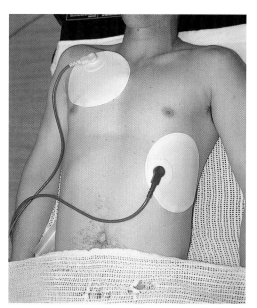

Electrode position for AED

Advantages of AEDs

The simplicity of operation of the AED has greatly reduced training requirements and extended the range of people that are able to provide defibrillation. The advent of the AED has allowed defibrillation by all grades of ambulance staff (not just specially trained paramedics) and in the United Kingdom the goal of equipping every emergency ambulance with a defibrillator has been achieved. Many other categories of healthcare professionals are able to defibrillate using an AED, and in most acute hospital wards and many other departments defibrillation can be undertaken by the staff present (usually nurses), well before the arrival of the cardiac arrest team.

It is almost impossible to deliver an inappropriate shock with an AED because the machine will only allow the operator to activate the appropriate control if an appropriate arrhythmia is detected. The operator, however, still has the responsibility for delivering the shock and for ensuring that everyone else is clear of the patient and safe before the charge is delivered.

Public access defibrillation

Conditions for defibrillation are often only optimal for as little as 90 seconds after the onset of defibrillation, and the need to reduce to a minimum the delay before delivery of a countershock has led to the development of novel ways of providing defibrillation. This is particularly so outside hospital where members of the public, rather than medical personnel, usually witness the event. The term "public access defibrillation" is used to describe the process by which defibrillation is performed by lay people trained in the use of an AED. These individuals (who are often staff working at places where the public congregate) operate within a system that is under medical control, but respond independently, usually on their own initiative, when someone collapses.

Early schemes to provide defibrillators in public places reported dramatic results. In the first year after their introduction at O'Hare airport, Chicago, several airline passengers who sustained a cardiac arrest were successfully resuscitated after defibrillation by staff at the airport. In Las Vegas, security staff at casinos have been trained to use AEDs with dramatic result; 56 out of 105 patients (53%) with VF survived to be discharged from hospital. The closed circuit TV surveillance in use at the casinos enabled rapid identification of potential patients, and 74% of those defibrillated within three minutes of collapsing survived.

Other locations where trained lay people undertake defibrillation are in aircraft and ships when a conventional response from the emergency services is impossible. In one report the cabin crew of American Airlines successfully

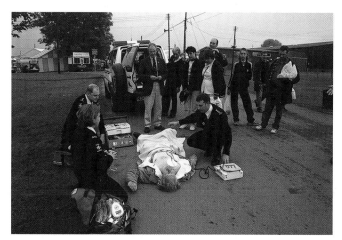

Defibrillation by first aiders

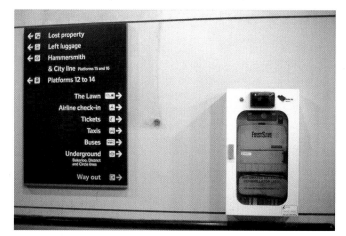

AED on a railway station

defibrillated all patients with VF, and 40% survived to leave hospital.

In the United Kingdom the remoteness of rural communities often prevents the ambulance service from responding quickly enough to a cardiac arrest or to the early stages of acute myocardial infarction. Increasingly, trained lay people (termed "first responders") living locally and equipped with an AED are dispatched by ambulance control at the same time as the ambulance itself. They are able to reach the patient and provide initial treatment, including defibrillation if necessary, before the ambulance arrives. Other strategies used to decrease response times include equipping the police and fire services with AEDs.

The provision of AEDs in large shopping complexes, airports, railway stations, and leisure facilities was introduced as government policy in England in 1999 as the "Defibrillators in Public Places" initiative. The British Heart Foundation has supported the concept of public access defibrillation enthusiastically and provided many defibrillators for use by trained lay responders working in organised schemes under the supervision of the ambulance service. As well as being used to treat patients who have collapsed, it is equally valid to apply an AED as a precautionary measure in people thought to be at risk of cardiac arrest—for example, in patients with chest pain. If cardiac arrest should subsequently occur, the rhythm will be analysed at the earliest opportunity, enabling defibrillation with the minimum delay.

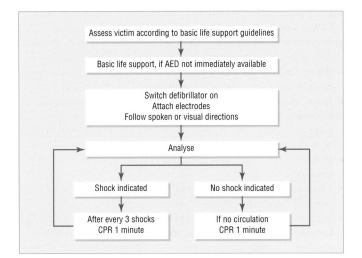

Algorithm for the use of AEDs

Sequence of actions with an AED

Once cardiac arrest has been confirmed it may be necessary for an assistant to perform basic life support while the equipment is prepared and the adhesive electrodes are attached to the patient's chest. The area of contact may need to be shaved if it is particularly hairy, and a small safety razor should be carried with the machine for this purpose.

The pulse or signs of a circulation should not be checked during delivery of each sequence of three shocks because this will interfere with the machine's analysis of the patient's ECG trace. Most machines have motion sensors that can detect any interference by a rescuer and will advise no contact between shocks.

Once the AED is ready to use, the following sequence should be used:

- Ensure safety of approach. If two rescuers are present one should go for help and to collect the AED while the other assesses the patient.
- Start CPR if the AED is not immediately available. Otherwise switch on the machine and apply the electrodes. One electrode should be placed at the upper right sternal border directly below the right clavicle. The other should be placed lateral to the left nipple with the top margin of the pad approximately 7 cm below the axilla. The correct position is usually indicated on the electrode packet or shown in a diagram on the AED itself. It may be necessary to dry the chest if the patient has been sweating noticeably or shave hair from the chest in the area where the pads are applied.
- Follow the voice prompts and visual directions. ECG analysis is usually performed automatically, but some machines require activation by pressing an "analyse" button.
- If a shock is indicated ensure that no one is in contact with the patient and shout "stand clear." Press the shock button once it is illuminated and the machine indicates it is ready to deliver the shock.

Safety factors

- All removable metal objects, such as chains and medallions, should be removed from the shock pathway—that is, from the front of the chest. Body jewellery that cannot be removed will need to be left in place. Although this may cause some minor skin burns in the immediate area, this risk has to be balanced against the delay involved in its removal
- Clothing should be open or cut to allow access to the patient's bare frontal chest area
- The patient's chest should be checked for the presence of self-medication patches on the front of the chest (these may deflect energy away from the heart)
- Oxygen that is being used—for example, with a pocket mask—should be directed away from the patient or turned off during defibrillation
- The environment should be checked for pools of water or metal surfaces that connect the patient to the operator. It is important to recognise that volatile atmospheres, such as petrol or aviation fumes, can ignite with a spark

Other factors

- Use screens to provide some dignity for the patient if members of the public are present
- Support may be required for people accompanying the casualty

- Repeat as directed for up to three shocks in any one sequence. Do not check for a pulse or other signs of a circulation between the three shocks.
- If no pulse or other sign of a circulation is found, perform CPR for one minute. This will be timed by the machine, after which it will prompt the operator to reanalyse the rhythm. Alternatively, this procedure may start automatically, depending on the machine's individual features or settings. Shocks should be repeated as indicated by the AED.
- If a circulation returns after a shock, check for breathing and continue to support the patient by rescue breathing if required. Check the patient every minute to ensure that signs of a circulation are still present.
- If the patient shows signs of recovery, place in the recovery position.
- Liaise with the emergency services when they arrive and provide full details of the actions undertaken.
- Report the incident to the medical supervisor in charge of the AED scheme so that data may be extracted from the machine. Ensure all supplies are replenished ready for the next use.

The diagram of the algorithm for the use of AEDs is adapted from *Resuscitation Guidelines 2000*, London: Resuscitation Council (UK), 2000.

Further reading

- Bossaert L, Koster R. Defibrillation methods and strategies. *Resuscitation* 1992;24:211-25.
- Cummins RO. From concept to standard of care? Review of the clinical experience with automated external defibrillators. *Ann Emerg Med* 1989;18:1269-76.
- Davies CS, Colquhoun MC, Graham S, Evans, T, Chamberlain D. Defibrillators in public places: the introduction of a national scheme for public access defibrillation in England. *Resuscitation* 2002;52:13-21.
- European Resuscitation Council Guidelines 2000 for automated defibrillation. *Resuscitation* 2001;48:207-9.
- International guidelines 2000 for cardiopulmonary resuscitation and cardiovascular emergency cardiac care—an international consensus on science. The automated defibrillator: key link in the chain of survival. *Resuscitation* 2000;46:73-91.
- International Advisory Group on Resuscitation ALS Working Group. The universal algorithm. *Resuscitation* 1997;34:109-11.
- Page RL, Joglar JA, Kowal RC, Zagrodsky JD, Nelson LL, Ramaswamy K, et al. Use of automated external defibrillators by a US airline. *N Eng J Med* 2000;343:1210-15.
- Resuscitation Council (UK). *Immediate life support manual.* London: Resuscitation Council (UK), 2002.
- Robertson CE, Steen P, Adjey J. European Resuscitation Council. Guidelines for adult advanced support. *Resuscitation* 1998;37:81-90.
- Valenzuela TD, Roe DJ, Nichol G, Clark LL, Spaite DW, Hardman RG. Outcomes of rapid defibrillation by security officers after cardiac arrest in casinos. *N Eng J Med* 2000;343:1206-9.

4 Asystole and pulseless electrical activity

Michael Colquhoun, A John Camm

Definition and epidemiology

Cardiac arrest can occur via three main mechanisms: ventricular fibrillation (VF), ventricular asystole, or pulseless electrical activity (PEA). PEA was formerly known as electromechanical dissociation but, by international agreement, PEA is now the preferred term.

In the community, VF is the commonest mode of cardiac arrest, particularly in patients with coronary disease, as described in Chapter 2. Asystole is the initial rhythm in about 10% of patients and PEA accounts for an even smaller proportion, probably less than 5%. The situation is different in hospital, where the primary mechanism of cardiac arrest is more often asystole or PEA. These rhythms are much more difficult to treat than VF and carry a much worse prognosis.

Asystolic cardiac arrest

Suppression of all natural or artificial cardiac pacemakers in asystolic cardiac arrest leads to ventricular standstill. Under normal circumstances an idioventricular rhythm will maintain cardiac output when either the supraventricular pacemakers fail or atrioventricular conduction is interrupted. Myocardial disease, electrolyte disturbance, anoxia, or drugs may suppress this idioventricular rhythm and cause asystole.

Excessive vagal activity may suddenly depress sinus or atrioventricular node function and cause asystole, especially when sympathetic tone is reduced—for example, by β blockers. Asystole will also occur as a terminal rhythm when VF is not successfully treated; the amplitude of the fibrillatory waveform declines progressively as myocardial energy and oxygen supplies are exhausted and asystole supervenes. When asystole occurs under these circumstances virtually no one survives. The chances of successful resuscitation are greater when asystole occurs at the onset of the arrest as the primary rhythm rather than as a secondary phenomenon.

Diagnosis and electrocardiographic appearances

Asystole is diagnosed when no activity can be seen on the electrocardiogram (ECG). Atrial and ventricular asystole usually coexist so that the ECG is a straight line with no recognisable deflections representing myocardial electrical activity. This straight line may, however, be distorted by baseline drift, electrical interference, respiratory movements, and artefacts arising from cardiopulmonary resuscitation (CPR). A completely straight line on the monitor screen often means that a monitoring lead has become disconnected.

VF may be mistaken for asystole if only one ECG lead is monitored or if the fibrillatory activity is of low amplitude. As VF is so readily treatable and resuscitation is more likely to be successful, it is vital that great care is taken before diagnosing asystole to the exclusion of VF. The electrocardiographic leads and their connections must all be checked, as must the gain and brilliance of the monitor. All contact with the patient should cease briefly to reduce the possibility of interference. An alternative ECG lead should be

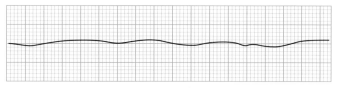

Asystole: baseline drift is present. The ECG is rarely a completely straight line in asystole

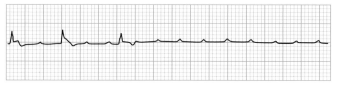

The onset of ventricular asystole complicating complete heart block

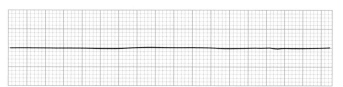

Onset of asystole due to sinoatrial block

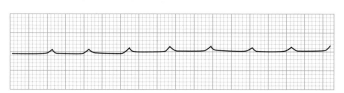

If the ECG appears as a straight line the leads, gain, and electrical connections must be checked

Ventricular asystole. Persistent P waves due to atrial depolarisation are seen recorded when the monitor has the facility to do this, or the defibrillator monitor electrodes should be moved to different positions.

On occasions, atrial activity may continue for a short time after the onset of ventricular asystole. In this case, the ECG will show a straight line interrupted by P waves but with no evidence of ventricular depolarisation.

PEA

Diagnosis

PEA is the term used to describe the features of cardiac arrest despite normal (or near normal) electrical excitation. The diagnosis is made from a combination of the clinical features of cardiac arrest in the presence of an ECG rhythm that would normally be accompanied by cardiac output.

The importance of recognising PEA is that it is often associated with specific clinical conditions that can be treated when PEA is promptly identified.

Causes

The causes of PEA can be divided into two broad categories. In "primary" PEA, excitation-contraction coupling fails, which results in a profound loss of cardiac output. Causes include massive myocardial infarction (particularly of the inferior wall), poisoning with drugs (for example, β blockers, calcium antagonists), or toxins, and electrolyte disturbance (hypocalcaemia, hyperkalaemia).

In "secondary" PEA, a mechanical barrier to ventricular filling or cardiac output exists. Causes include tension pneumothorax, pericardial tamponade, cardiac rupture, pulmonary embolism, occlusion of a prosthetic heart valve, and hypovolaemia. These are summarised in the 4Hs/4Ts mnemonic (see base of algorithm). Treatment in all cases is directed towards the underlying cause.

Management of asystole and PEA

Guidelines for the treatment of cardiopulmonary arrest caused by asystole or PEA are contained in the universal advanced life support algorithm.

Treatment for all cases of cardiac arrest is determined by the presence or absence of a rhythm likely to respond to a countershock. In the absence of a shockable rhythm "non-VF/VT" is diagnosed. This category includes all patients with asystole or PEA. Both are treated in the same way, by following the right-hand side of the algorithm.

When using a manual defibrillator and ECG monitor, non-VF/VT will be recognised by the clinical appearance of the patient and the rhythm on the monitor screen. When using an automated defibrillator, non-VF/VT rhythms are diagnosed when the machine dictates that no shock is indicated and the patient has no signs of a circulation. When the rhythm is checked on a monitor screen, the ECG trace should be examined carefully for the presence of P waves or other electrical activity that may respond to cardiac pacing. Pacing is often effective when applied to patients with asystole due to atrioventricular block or failure of sinus node discharge. It is unlikely to be successful when asystole follows extensive myocardial impairment or systemic metabolic upset. The role of cardiac pacing in the management of patients with cardiopulmonary arrest is considered further in Chapter 17.

As soon as a non-VF/VT rhythm is diagnosed, basic life support should be performed for three minutes, after which the rhythm should be reassessed. During this first loop of the

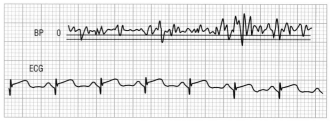

Pulseless electrical activity in a patient with acute myocardial infarction. Despite an apparently near normal cardiac rhythm there was no blood pressure (BP)

> PEA can be a primary cardiac event or secondary to a potentially reversible disorder

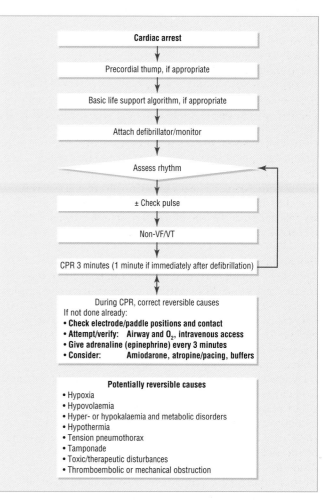

The advanced life support algorithm for the management of non-VF cardiac arrest in adults. Adapted from *Resuscitation Guidelines 2000*, London: Resuscitation Council (UK), 2000

algorithm, the airway may be secured, intravenous access obtained, and the first dose of adrenaline (epinephrine) given. If asystole is present atropine, in a single dose of 3 mg intravenously (6 mg by tracheal tube), should be given to block the vagus nerve completely.

The best chance of resuscitation from asystole or PEA occurs when a secondary, treatable cause is responsible for the arrest. For this reason the search for such a cause assumes major importance. The most common treatable causes are listed as the 4Hs and 4Ts at the foot of the universal algorithm. Loops of the right-hand side of the algorithm are repeated, with further doses of adrenaline (epinephrine) given every three minutes while the search for an underlying cause is made and treatment instigated.

If, during the treatment of asystole or PEA, the rhythm changes to VF (which will be evident on a monitor screen or by an automated external defibrillator advising that a shock is indicated) then the left-hand side of the universal algorithm should be followed with attempts at defibrillation.

Asystole after defibrillation

If asystole or PEA occurs immediately after the delivery of a shock, CPR should be administered but the rhythm and circulation should be checked after only one minute before any further drugs are given. This procedure is recommended because a temporarily poor cardiac output due to myocardial stunning after defibrillation may result in an impalpable pulse and a spurious diagnosis. After one minute of CPR the cardiac output might improve and the presence of a circulation becomes apparent. In this situation further adrenaline (epinephrine) could be detrimental, and this recommended procedure is designed to avoid this.

If asystole or PEA is confirmed, the appropriate drugs should be administered and a further two minutes of CPR are given to complete the loop.

Spurious asystole may also occur after the delivery of a shock when monitoring is conducted through the defibrillator electrodes using gel defibrillator pads. This becomes increasingly likely when a number of shocks have been delivered through the same gel pads. Monitoring with the defibrillator electrodes is unreliable in this situation and a diagnosis of asystole should be confirmed independently by conventional electrocardiograph monitoring leads.

4Hs

● Hypoxia
● Hypovolaemia
● Hyper- or hypokalaemia and metabolic causes
● Hypothermia

4Ts

● Tension pneumothorax
● Tamponade
● Toxic or therapeutic disturbance
● Thromboembolic or mechanical

After the delivery of a shock, it takes a few moments before the monitor display recovers; during this time the rhythm may be interpreted erroneously as asystole. With modern defibrillators this period is relatively short but it is important to be aware of the potential problem, particularly with older equipment

Gel defibrillator pads may cause spurious asystole to be seen because they are able to act like a capacitor and store small quantities of electrical charge sufficient to mask the electrical activity from the heart

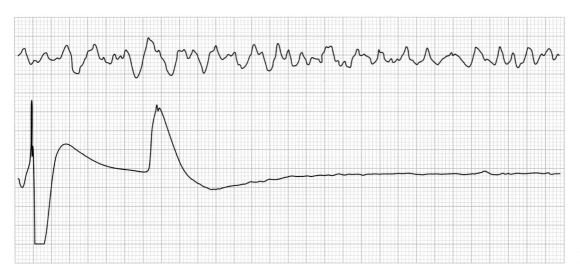

Asystole after defibrillation

Drug treatments

Atropine is recommended in the treatment of cardiac arrest due to asystole or PEA to block fully the effects of possible vagal overactivity; its use in this role is considered further in Chapter 16. In the past, calcium, alkalising agents, high dose adrenaline (epinephrine), and other pressor drugs have been employed, but little evidence is available to justify their use and none are included in current treatment guidelines. These are also considered in Chapter 16.

Interest has recently been focused on a possible role of adenosine antagonists in the treatment of asystolic cardiac arrest. Myocardial ischaemia is a potent stimulus for the release of adenosine, which then accumulates in the myocardium and slows the heart rate by suppressing cardiac automaticity; it may also produce atrioventricular block. Adenosine attenuates β adrenergic mediated increases in myocardial contractility and may increase coronary blood flow. Although these effects may be cardioprotective, it has been suggested that under some circumstances they may produce or maintain cardiac asystole.

Aminophylline and other methylxanthines act as adenosine receptor blocking agents, and anecdotal accounts of successful resuscitation from asystole after their use have led to more detailed investigation. A pilot study reported encouraging results but subsequent small studies have not shown such dramatic results nor any clear benefit from the use of aminophylline. There may be a subgroup of patients who would benefit greatly from adenosine receptor blockade but at present they cannot be identified. The use of aminophylline is not included in current resuscitation guidelines and its use in the treatment of asystole remains empirical pending further evidence.

Further reading

- European Resuscitation Council. European Resuscitation Council guidelines 2000 for adult advanced life support. *Resuscitation* 2001;48:211-21.
- International guidelines 2000 for cardiopulmonary resuscitation and emergency cardiovascular care—an international consensus on science. Part 6: advanced cardiovascular life support. *Resuscitation* 2000;46:169-84.
- Mader TJ, Smithline HA, Gibson P. Aminophylline in undifferentiated out-of-hospital cardiac arrest. *Resuscitation* 1999; 41:39-45.
- Viskin S, Belhassen B, Berne R. Aminophylline for bradysystolic cardiac arrest refractory to atropine and epinephrine. *Ann Intern Med* 1993;118:279-81.

5 Management of peri-arrest arrhythmias

Michael Colquhoun, Richard Vincent

A coordinated strategy to reduce death from cardiac arrest should include not only cardiopulmonary resuscitation but also measures to treat potentially malignant arrhythmias that may lead to cardiac arrest or complicate the period after resuscitation. The term "peri-arrest arrhythmia" is used to describe such a cardiac rhythm disturbance in this situation.

Cardiac arrest should be prevented wherever possible by the effective treatment of warning arrhythmias. Ventricular fibrillation is often triggered by ventricular tachycardia and asystole may complicate progressive bradycardia or complete heart block. Malignant rhythm disturbances may also complicate the post-resuscitation period and effective treatment will greatly improve the patient's chance of survival.

Staff who provide the initial management of patients with cardiopulmonary arrest are not usually trained in the management of complex arrhythmias, and the peri-arrest arrhythmia guidelines are designed to tackle this situation. The European Resuscitation Council (ERC) first published guidelines for the management of peri-arrest arrhythmias in 1994. These were revised in 2001, based on the evidence review undertaken in preparation for the *International Guidelines 2000*. The recommendations are intended to be straightforward in their application and, as far as possible, applicable in all European countries, not withstanding their different traditions of anti-arrhythmic treatment.

The guidelines offer advice on the appropriate treatment that might be expected from any individual trained in the immediate management of cardiac arrest. They also indicate when expert help should be sought and offer suggestions for more advanced strategies when such help is not immediately available.

Four categories of rhythm disturbance are considered and the recommended treatments for each are summarised in the form of an algorithm. The first algorithm covers the treatment of bradycardia, defined as a ventricular rate of less than 60 beats/min. Two further algorithms summarise the treatment of patients with tachycardia, defined as a ventricular rate of greater than 100 beats/min. The two tachycardia algorithms are distinguished by the width of the QRS complex. A "narrow complex tachycardia" is defined as a QRS duration of 100 msec or less, whereas a "broad complex tachycardia" has a QRS complex of greater than 100 milliseconds. Finally, an algorithm has been developed for the treatment of atrial fibrillation.

The principles of treatment for peri-arrest arrhythmias are similar to those used in other clinical contexts but the following points deserve emphasis:

- The algorithms are designed specifically for the peri-arrest situation and are not intended to encompass all clinical situations in which such arrhythmias may be encountered.
- In all cases, treatment is determined by clinical assessment of the patient and not by the electrocardiographic appearances alone.
- The algorithms are intended for clinicians who do not regard themselves as experts in the management of arrhythmias.

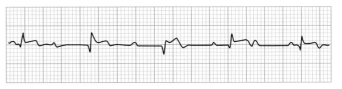

Complete heart block complicating inferior infarction: narrow QRS complex

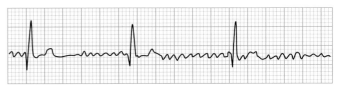

Atrial fibrillation with complete heart block. Bradycardia may arise for many reasons. Assessment of the cardiac output is essential

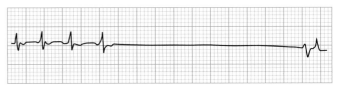

Asystole lasting 2.5 seconds due to sinoatrial block

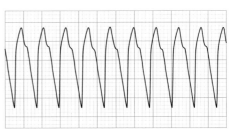

Antidromic atrioventricular re-entrant tachycardia

- The arrows in the algorithms that indicate progression from one treatment stage to the next are only followed if the arrhythmia persists.
- All anti-arrhythmic strategies (whether physical manoeuvres, drugs, or electrical treatment) may have pro-arrhythmic effects. Therefore, remember that deterioration of the patient's condition may be the result of treatment rather than its lack of efficacy.
- The pro-arrhythmic effects of anti-arrhythmic drugs become potentially greater hazards when more than one drug is used. The use of more than one anti-arrhythmic drug in any situation is a matter for very skilled judgement.
- The use of multiple anti-arrhythmic drugs or high doses of a single agent may cause myocardial depression and hypotension. The extent to which sequential treatment should be carried out in the face of these risks will be a matter for skilled clinical judgement.
- The algorithms include doses based on average body weight and may need adjustment in specific cases.

Bradycardias

Bradycardia is defined as a ventricular rate below 60 beats/min. However, it is important to recognise the patient whose heart rate, although greater than 60 beats/min, may be inappropriately slow for their haemodynamic state.

If any of these signs are present, atropine (500 mcg intravenously) should be given. If this is successful, subsequent treatment should be governed by the presence or absence of risk factors for asystole (see below). If atropine is unsuccessful, however, further doses of 500 mcg may be given up to a maximum of 3 mg. Transcutaneous/external pacing should be used if equipment is available. If atropine is unsuccessful and if external pacing is not available, a low dose adrenaline (epinephrine) infusion is recommended; isoprenaline is no longer advocated. All these measures must be regarded as holding procedures until temporary transvenous pacing can be established.

In the absence of adverse signs, or after successful treatment with 500 mcg atropine, further intervention is only justified if the patient is thought to be at high risk of asystole. Factors that suggest this are a previous history of asystole, Möbitz type 2 atrioventricular (AV) block, complete heart block with a wide QRS complex, or ventricular pauses greater than three seconds. If any of these factors are present, further atropine should be given, or external pacing instituted while temporary transvenous pacing is being arranged. If no adverse signs are present, and the patient is not at risk of asystole, the patient should simply be observed closely.

Tachycardia

Tachyarrhythmias are conventionally divided into those arising within the ventricular myocardium (ventricular tachycardias) or those arising above, or sometimes within, the AV junction (supraventricular tachycardias). This has obvious merit with regard to treatment and prognosis, but considerable diagnostic difficulties may be encountered when relating the electrocardiographic appearance to the underlying mechanism of an arrhythmia.

Ventricular tachycardia characteristically has a broad width QRS complex, but some rare tachycardias arising below the

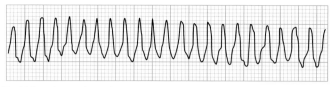

Rapid broad complex tachycardia: if the patient is unconscious, without a pulse, treatment is the same as for ventricular fibrillation

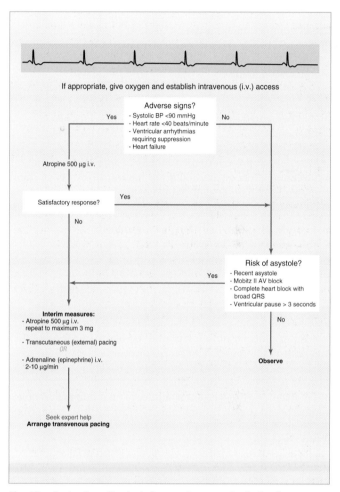

If appropriate, give oxygen and establish intravenous (i.v.) access

Adverse signs?
- Systolic BP <90 mmHg
- Heart rate <40 beats/minute
- Ventricular arrhythmias requiring suppression
- Heart failure

Atropine 500 µg i.v.

Satisfactory response? — Yes

Risk of asystole?
- Recent asystole
- Mobitz II AV block
- Complete heart block with broad QRS
- Ventricular pause > 3 seconds

Interim measures:
- Atropine 500 µg i.v. repeat to maximum 3 mg
- Transcutaneous (external) pacing
  OR
- Adrenaline (epinephrine) i.v. 2-10 µg/min

Observe

Seek expert help
Arrange transvenous pacing

Algorithm for bradycardia—includes rates inappropriately slow for haemodynamic state. Adapted from *ALS Course Provider Manual.* 4th ed. London: Resuscitation Council (UK), 2000

Certain adverse signs in bradycardia dictate the need for intervention:

- Systolic blood pressure less than 90 mmHg
- Ventricular rate less than 40 beats/min
- Presence of ventricular arrhythmias requiring treatment
- Presence of heart failure

AV junction may have a complex width within the normal range. Supraventricular tachycardia characteristically has a narrow QRS, but it may be widened when conduction is abnormal—for example, in the presence of bundle branch block. The guidelines make no assumption that the mechanism of tachycardia has been accurately defined and the recommendations for treatment are based on a simple electrocardiogram classification into narrow or broad complex tachycardia. In the context of peri-arrest arrhythmia, it is always safest to assume that a broad complex tachycardia is ventricular in origin.

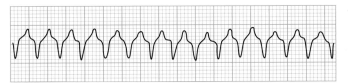

Broad complex tachycardia: treatment will depend on the presence of adverse signs

Broad complex tachycardia

Little harm results if supraventricular tachycardia is treated as a ventricular arrhythmia; however, the converse error may have serious consequences.

The first question that determines management is whether a palpable pulse is present. Pulseless ventricular tachycardia should be treated as cardiac arrest using the ventricular fibrillation or pulseless ventricular tachycardia protocols described in Chapter 2.

If a pulse is present oxygen should be administered and intravenous access established if this has not already been done. Treatment will then be determined by the presence or absence of adverse signs. The algorithm describes four such signs:

- A systolic blood pressure less than 90 mmHg.
- The presence of chest pain.
- The presence of heart failure.
- A ventricular rate of more than 150 beats/min.

If any of these signs are present the situation should be regarded as an emergency and cardioversion, under appropriate sedation, should be attempted. If the plasma potassium concentration is known to be less than 3.6 mmol/l, especially in the presence of recent myocardial infarction, an infusion of potassium and magnesium is recommended (according to the algorithm) before cardioversion is undertaken. If cardioversion is unsuccessful it is appropriate to administer an anti-arrhythmic agent before further attempts are made; amiodarone is considered the agent of first choice. If these measures are unsuccessful additional doses of amiodarone or alternative anti-arrhythmic drugs may be considered, preferably given under expert guidance. Overdrive pacing may be a useful strategy in this situation if the necessary expertise is available.

In the absence of adverse signs the situation is less urgent. If the serum potassium concentration is known to be low an infusion of potassium and magnesium should be given. If the potassium concentration is unknown it must be measured immediately. Amiodarone is again recommended as the drug of first choice to stop the tachycardia; lignocaine (lidocaine) remains an alternative. With most patients there should be time to consult expert help to advise about management. Synchronised cardioversion should preferably be attempted after allowing one hour for the amiodarone infusion to take effect. If cardioversion is initially unsuccessful further doses of amiodarone should be given, allowing time for the drug's powerful anti-arrhythmic action before cardioversion is repeated.

Should the patient's condition deteriorate and adverse signs develop, immediate electrical cardioversion should be undertaken.

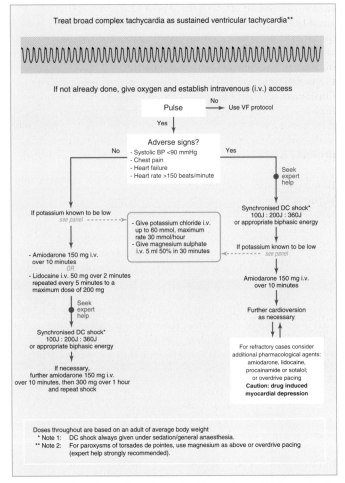

Algorithm for broad complex tachycardia. Adapted from *ALS Course Provider Manual*. 4th ed. London: Resuscitation Council (UK), 2000

Overdrive pacing is a technique whereby the heart is paced for a limited period at a rate higher than the tachycardia. The tachycardia may be abolished with a return of normal rhythm when the pacemaker is switched off

Narrow complex tachycardia

A narrow complex tachycardia is virtually always supraventricular in origin—that is, the activating impulse of the tachycardia passes through the AV node. Supraventricular tachycardias are, in general, less dangerous than those of ventricular origin and only rarely occur after the successful treatment of ventricular tachyarrhythmias. Nevertheless, they are a recognised trigger for the development of ventricular fibrillation in vulnerable patients.

If the patient is pulseless in association with a narrow complex tachycardia, then electrical cardioversion should be attempted immediately. As in the treatment of any serious rhythm disturbance, oxygen should be administered and intravenous access established.

At this stage it is important to exclude the presence of atrial fibrillation. This is a common arrhythmia occurring before cardiac arrest and often in the post-resuscitation period. In atrial fibrillation the ventricular response is irregular, unlike the regular ventricular pattern seen with other rhythms that arise above the AV junction. At faster ventricular rates it may be difficult to determine whether the rhythm is regular because the variation in the R-R interval, which is a feature of atrial fibrillation, becomes less pronounced. Atrial fibrillation may then seem to be regular and the distinction can only be made if an adequate rhythm strip is examined carefully for variability in the underlying rate. Guidance to treat atrial fibrillation is provided in the next section and accompanying algorithm.

Regular narrow complex tachycardia

Vagotonic manoeuvres, such as the Valsava manoeuvre or carotid sinus massage, should always be considered as first line treatment. Caution is required, however, as profound vagal tone may cause a sudden bradycardia and trigger ventricular fibrillation, particularly in the presence of acute ischaemia or digitalis toxicity. Carotid sinus massage may result in rupture of an atheromatous plaque and the possibility of a stroke.

The drug of choice for the initial treatment of regular supraventricular tachycardia is adenosine 6 mg by rapid bolus injection. If this is unsuccessful up to three further doses of 12 mg may be given, allowing one to two minutes between injections. If adenosine fails to convert the rhythm, then expert help should be sought and the patient checked carefully for the presence of adverse signs.

In the presence of one or more of these adverse signs treatment should consist of synchronised DC cardioversion after appropriate sedation. If this is unsuccessful a further attempt at cardioversion should be made after a slow intravenous injection and subsequent infusion of amiodarone. If circumstances permit, up to one hour should be allowed for the drug to exert its anti-arrhythmic effect before further attempts at cardioversion are made.

In the absence of adverse signs there is no single recommendation in the ERC Guidelines for the treatment of persistent narrow complex tachycardia because of the different traditions between European countries. The suggestions offered include a short acting β blocker (esmolol), a calcium channel blocking agent (verapamil), digoxin, or amiodarone. Verapamil is widely used in this situation, but it is important to remember that there are several contra-indications. These include arrhythmias associated with the Wolff-Parkinson-White syndrome, tachycardias that are, in fact, ventricular in origin, and some of the childhood supraventricular arrhythmias. A potentially serious interaction may occur between verapamil and β adrenergic blocking agents; this is particularly likely to happen if both drugs have been administered intravenously.

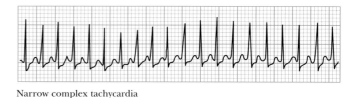

Narrow complex tachycardia

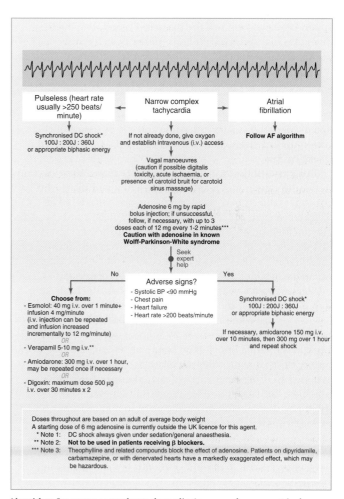

Algorithm for narrow complex tachycardia (presumed supraventricular tachycardia). Adapted from *ALS Course Provider Manual.* 4th ed. London: Resuscitation council (UK), 2000

Regular narrow complex tachycardia: adverse signs

- A systolic blood pressure less than 90 mmHg
- The presence of chest pain
- Heart failure
- A heart rate greater than 200 beats/min

Atrial fibrillation

In atrial fibrillation all coordination of atrial systole is lost and ventricular filling during diastole becomes a passive process. The orderly control of ventricular rate and rhythm that exists during normal sinus rhythm is lost and the ventricular rate is determined by the refractory period of the AV node. When this is short a rapid ventricular rate may result, which further reduces cardiac output.

The treatment of atrial fibrillation centres on three key objectives: to control ventricular rate, to restore sinus rhythm, and to prevent systemic embolism.

Thrombus forms in the left atrium, particularly in the atrial appendage, as a result of the disturbed blood flow. Such thrombus may form within hours of the onset of atrial fibrillation and the risk of embolisation is particularly great at the point that sinus rhythm is restored. The need for anticoagulation to reduce this risk fundamentally influences the approach to treatment of this arrhythmia.

Patients may be placed into one of three risk groups depending on the ventricular rate and the presence of clinical symptoms and signs. The treatment of each is summarised in the algorithm.

Patients with a ventricular rate greater than 150 beats/min, those with ongoing ischaemic cardiac pain, and those who have critically reduced peripheral perfusion are considered at particularly high risk. Immediate anticoagulation with heparin and an attempt at cardioversion is recommended. This should be followed by an infusion of amiodarone to maintain sinus rhythm if it has been restored, or control ventricular rate in situations in which atrial fibrillation persists or recurs.

Patients with a ventricular rate of less than 100 beats/min, with no symptoms, and good peripheral perfusion constitute a low risk group. When the onset of atrial fibrillation is known to have been within the previous 24 hours anticoagulation with heparin should be undertaken before an attempt is made to restore sinus rhythm, either by pharmacological or electrical means. Two drugs are suggested, amiodarone or flecainide, which are both given by intravenous infusion. Only one drug should be used in an individual patient to minimise the risk of pro-arrhythmic effects and myocardial depression. DC cardioversion may be attempted, either as a first line treatment to restore sinus rhythm, or when pharmacological efforts have been unsuccessful. If atrial fibrillation is of longer standing (more than 24 hours) the decision to attempt to restore sinus rhythm should be made after careful clinical assessment, taking into account the chances of achieving and maintaining a normal rhythm. The majority of patients in this group will require initial anticoagulation with heparin while treatment with warfarin is stabilised. Elective cardioversion should not be attempted before the patient has been anticoagulated for three to four weeks.

The two groups of patients discussed so far represent the two extremes of risk posed by atrial fibrillation. An additional group at intermediate risk is classified on the basis of a heart rate of 100-150 beats/min. This group poses a difficult challenge for treatment and in all cases expert help should be consulted if available. Further management depends on the presence or absence of poor peripheral perfusion or structural heart disease. Treatment depends on the length of time that fibrillation has been present. If this is less than 24 hours, the patient should receive immediate anticoagulation with heparin followed by an attempt at cardioversion, either using drugs (amiodarone or flecainide) or electrically. If fibrillation has been present for more than 24 hours, heparin and warfarin should be started and elective cardioversion considered once the oral anticoagulation has been stabilised (international normalised ratio 2-3) for three to four weeks.

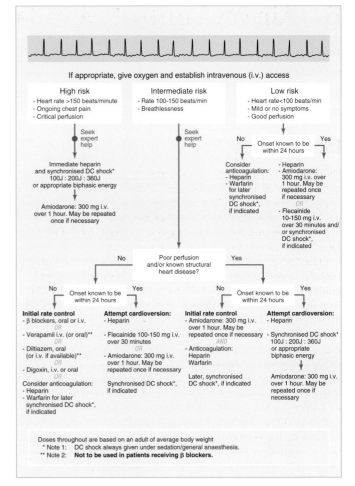

Algorithm for atrial fibrillation (presumed supraventricular tachycardia). Adapted from *ALS Course Provider Manual*. 4th ed. London: Resuscitation Council (UK), 2000

If cardioversion proves impossible or atrial fibrillation recurs, amiodarone will provide ventricular rate control. It is also a useful drug to increase the chances of successful cardioversion in patients with adverse features such as poor left ventricular function.

Further reading

- Chamberlain DA. The periarrest arrhythmias. *Br J Anaesthesia* 1997;79:198-202.
- Dorian P, Cass D, Schwartz B Cooper R, Gelaznikas R, Bara A. Amiodarone as compared with lidocaine for shock resistant ventricular fibrillation (ALIVE). *N Engl J Med* 2002;34:884-90.
- European Resuscitation Council. European resuscitation council guidelines for adult advanced life support. *Resuscitation* 2001;48:211-21.
- International guidelines 2000 for cardiopulmonary resuscitation and emergency cardiac care—an international consensus on science. Section 5: agents for arrhythmias. *Resuscitation* 2000;46:135-53; Section 7C A guide to the international ACLS algorithms. *Resuscitation* 2000;46:169-84; Section 7D The tachycardia algorithms. *Resuscitation* 2000;46: 185-93.
- Kudenchuk PJ, Cobb LA, Copass MK, Cummins RO, Doherty AM, Farenbruch CE, et al. Amiodarone for resuscitation after out-of-hospital cardiac arrest due to ventricular fibrillation (ARREST). *N Engl J Med* 1999;341:871-8.

6 Airway control, ventilation, and oxygenation

Robert Simons

Introduction

Oxidative cellular metabolism requires a constant consumption of oxygen by all organs, amounting to 250 ml/min in a typical adult. This necessitates both an unobstructed bellows action by the lungs to replace oxygen and eliminate carbon dioxide in the gas phase, and a continuous pulsatile action by the heart for effective delivery of the blood to the tissues.

The "oxygen cascade" described by J B West 35 years ago explains how oxygen is conducted down a series of tension gradients from the atmosphere to cellular mitochondria. These "supply and demand" gradients increase when disease states or trauma interfere with the normal oxygen flux. Partial or total reduction of ventilation or blood flow are obvious examples and form the fundamental basis for the ABC of resuscitation. Other subtle causes coexist. Within the lung parenchyma at alveolar level, ventilation (V) and pulmonary artery perfusion (Q) are optimally matched to maintain an efficient V/Q ratio such that neither wasted ventilation (dead-space effect) nor wasted perfusion (shunt effect) occurs.

Medical conditions and trauma—for example, aspiration, pneumonia, sepsis, haemorrhage, pneumothorax, pulmonary haematoma, and myocardial damage caused by infarction or injury—can severely impair pulmonary gas exchange and result in arterial desaturation. This causes hypoxaemia (low blood oxygen tension and reduced oxyhaemoglobin saturation). The resulting clinical cyanosis may pass unrecognised in poor ambient light conditions and in black patients. The use of pulse oximetry (SpO_2) monitoring during resuscitation is recommended but requires pulsatile blood flow to function. A combination of arterial hypoxaemia and impaired arterial oxygen delivery (causing myocardial damage, acute blood loss, or severe anaemia) may render vital organs reversibly or irreversibly hypoxic. The brain will respond with loss of consciousness, risking (further) obstructed ventilation or unprotected pulmonary aspiration (or both). Impaired oxygen supply to the heart may affect contractility and induce rhythm disturbances if not already present. Renal and gut hypoxaemia do not usually present immediate problems but may contribute to "multiple organ dysfunction" at a later stage.

Airway patency

Failure to maintain a patent airway is a recognised cause of avoidable death in unconscious patients. The principles of airway management during cardiac arrest or after major trauma are the same as those during anaesthesia.

Airway patency may be impaired by the loss of normal muscle tone or by obstruction. In the unconscious patient relaxation of the tongue, neck, and pharyngeal muscles causes soft tissue obstruction of the supraglottic airway. This may be corrected by the techniques of head tilt with jaw lift or jaw thrust. The use of head tilt will relieve obstruction in 80% of patients but should not be used if a cervical spine injury is suspected. Chin lift or jaw thrust will further improve airway patency but will tend to oppose the lips. With practice, chin lift

---

Normal ventilation of a 70 kg adult comprises:

- A respiratory minute volume of 6 l/min air containing 21% oxygen, with a tidal volume of 500 ml at 12 breaths/min
- An expired oxygen level of 16-17%, hence its use in expired air resuscitation
- Cardiac output is typically 5 l/min at 60-80 beats/min. In the presence of a normal haemoglobin level and arterial oxygen saturation above 94%, this amounts to an oxygen availability of 1000 ml/min
- Average tissue oxygen extraction is only 25%, thereby providing reserves for increased oxygen extraction during exercise, disease, or trauma where oxygen delivery is impaired

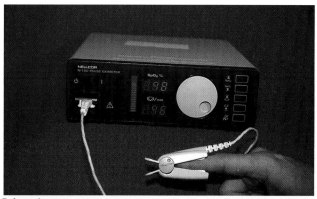

Pulse oximeter

"A secure airway and ventilation with oxygen remains the gold standard for ventilation in patients requiring assisted ventilation"
Wenzel et al (2001)

The ABC philosophy in both cardiac and trauma life support relies on a combination of actions to achieve airway patency, optimal ventilation, and cardiac output, and to restore and maintain circulatory blood volume

and jaw thrust can be performed without causing cervical spine movement. In some patients, airway obstruction may be particularly noticeable during expiration, due to the flap-valve effect of the soft palate against the nasopharyngeal tissues, which occurs in snoring. Obstruction may also occur by contamination from material in the mouth, nasopharynx, oesophagus, or stomach—for example, food, vomit, blood, chewing gum, foreign bodies, broken teeth or dentures, blood, or weed during near-drowning.

Laryngospasm (adductor spasm of the vocal cords) is one of the most primitive and potent animal reflexes. It results from stimuli to, or the presence of foreign material in, the oro- and laryngopharynx and may ironically occur after cardiac resuscitation as the brain stem reflexes are re-established.

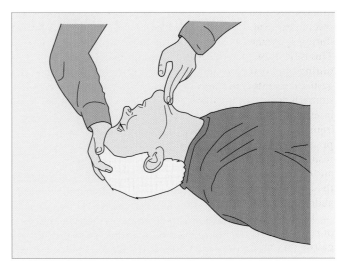

Airway patency maintained by the head tilt/chin lift

Recovery posture

Patients with adequate spontaneous ventilation and circulation who cannot safeguard their own airway will be at risk of developing airway obstruction in the supine position. Turning the patient into the recovery position allows the tongue to fall forward, with less risk of pharyngeal obstruction, and fluid in the mouth can then drain outwards instead of soiling the trachea and lungs. This is described in Chapter 1.

Spinal injury

The casualty with suspected spinal injuries requires careful handling and should be managed supine, with the head and cervical spine maintained in the neutral anatomical position; constant attention is needed to ensure that the airway remains patent. The head and neck should be maintained in a neutral position using a combination of manual inline immobilisation, a semi-rigid collar, sandbags, spinal board, and securing straps. The usual semi-prone recovery position should not be used because considerable rotation of the neck is required to prevent the casualty lying on his or her face. If a casualty must be turned, he or she should be "log rolled" into a true lateral position by several rescuers in unison, taking care to avoid rotation or flexion of the spine, especially the cervical spine. If the head or upper chest is injured, bony neck injury should be assumed to be present until excluded by lateral cervical spine radiography and examination by a specialist. Further management of the airway in patients in whom trauma to the cervical spine is suspected is provided in Chapter 14.

Casualties with spinal injury often develop significant gastric atony and dilation, and may require nasogastric aspiration or cricoid pressure to prevent gastric aspiration and tracheobronchial soiling.

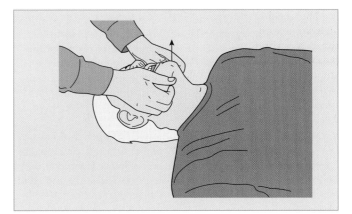

Airway patency maintained by jaw thrust

Vomiting and regurgitation

Rescuers should always be alert to the risk of contamination of the unprotected airway by regurgitation or vomiting of fluid or solid debris. Impaired consciousness from anaesthesia, head injury, hypoxia, centrally depressant drugs (opioids and recreational drugs), and circulatory depression or arrest will rapidly impair the cough and gag reflexes that normally prevent tracheal soiling.

Vomiting is an active process of stomach contraction with retrograde propulsion up the oesophagus. It occurs more commonly during lighter levels of unconsciousness or when cerebral perfusion improves after resuscitation from cardiac arrest. Prodromal retching may allow time to place the patient in the lateral recovery position or head down (Trendelenburg) tilt, and prepare for suction or manual removal of debris from the mouth and pharynx.

Regurgitation is a passive, often silent, flow of stomach contents (typically fluid) up the oesophagus, with the risk of

Medical conditions affecting the cough and gag reflexes include:

- Cerebrovascular accidents
- Bulbar and cranial nerve palsies
- Guillain-Barré syndrome
- Demyelinating disorders
- Motor neurone disease
- Myasthenia gravis

inhalation and soiling of the lungs. Acid gastric fluid may cause severe chemical pneumonitis. Failure to maintain a clear airway during spontaneous ventilation may encourage regurgitation. This is because negative intrathoracic pressure developed during obstructed inspiration may encourage aspiration of gastric contents across a weak mucosal flap valve between the stomach and oesophagus. Recent food or fluid ingestion, intestinal obstruction, recent trauma (especially spinal cord injury or in children), obesity, hiatus hernia, and late pregnancy all make regurgitation more likely to occur. During resuscitation, chest compression over the lower sternum and/or abdominal thrusts (no longer recommended) increase the likelihood of regurgitation as well as risking damage to the abdominal organs.

Gaseous distension of the stomach increases the likelihood of regurgitation and restricts chest expansion. Inadvertent gastric distension may occur during assisted ventilation, especially if large tidal volumes and high inflation pressures are used. This is particularly likely to happen if laryngospasm is present or when gas-powered resuscitators are used in conjunction with facemasks.

The cricoid pressure, or Sellick manoeuvre, is performed by an assistant and entails compression of the oesophagus between the cricoid ring and the sixth cervical vertebra to prevent passive regurgitation. It must not be applied during active vomiting, which could provoke an oesophageal tear.

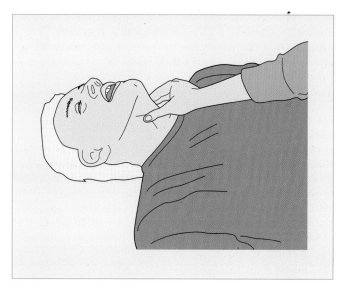

Sellick manoeuvre of cricoid pressure

Choking

Asphyxia due to impaction of food or other foreign body in the upper airway is a dramatic and frightening event. In the conscious patient back blows and thoracic thrusts (the modified Heimlich manoeuvre) have been widely recommended. If respiratory obstruction persists, the patient will become unconscious and collapse. The supine patient may be given further thoracic thrusts, and manual attempts at pharyngeal disimpaction should be undertaken. Visual inspection of the throat with a laryngoscope and the use of Magill forceps or suction is desirable.

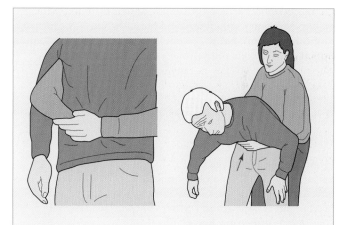

Abdominal thrust

Suction

Equipment for suction clearance of the oropharynx is essential for the provision of comprehensive life support. When choosing one of the many devices available, considerations of cost, portability, and power supply are paramount. Devices powered by electricity or compressed gas risk exhaustion of the power supply at a critical time; battery operated devices require regular recharging or battery replacement. Hand or foot operated pumps are particularly suitable for field use and suit the occasional user. Ease of cleaning and reassembly are important factors when choosing such a device. A rigid, wide bore metal or plastic suction cannula can be supplemented by the use of soft plastic suction catheters when necessary. A suction booster that traps fluid debris in a reservoir close to the patient may improve the suction capability.

> If attempts at relieving choking are unsuccessful, the final hypoxic event may be indistinguishable from other types of cardiac arrest. Treatment should follow the ABC (airway, breathing, and circulation) routine, although ventilation may be difficult or impossible to perform. The act of chest compression may clear the offending object from the laryngopharynx

Surgical intervention: needle and surgical cricothyrotomy

In situations in which the vocal cords remain obstructed—for example, by a foreign body, maxillofacial trauma, extrinsic pressure, or inflammation—and the patient can neither self-ventilate nor be ventilated using the airway adjuncts discussed below, urgent recourse to needle jet ventilation or surgical cricothyrotomy, or both, should be considered.

Narrow-bore oxygen tubing connected to a wall or cylinder flowmeter supplying oxygen up to 4 bar/60 p.s.i. can be pushed into a syringe barrel and attached to a 12-14 gauge needle or cannula inserted through the cricothyroid membrane. A hole cut in the oxygen tubing enables finger tip control of ventilation. Minimise barotrauma or pneumothorax by maintaining a one second:four second inflation to exhalation cycle to allow adequate time for expiration. A second open transcricoid needle or cannula may facilitate expiration but spontaneous ventilation by this route will be inadequate and strenuous inspiratory efforts will rapidly induce pulmonary oedema. Beware of jet needle displacement resulting in obstruction, gastric distension, pharyngeal or mediastinal perforation, and surgical emphysema.

Jet ventilation can maintain reasonable oxygenation for up to 45 minutes despite rising CO_2 levels until a cricothrotomy or definitive tracheostomy can be performed. If needle jet ventilation is unavailable or is ineffective, cricothyrotomy may be life saving and should not be unduly delayed. In the absence of surgical instruments any strong knife, scissors point, large bore cannula, or similar instrument can be used to create an opening through the cricothyroid membrane. An opening of 5-7 mm diameter is made and needs to be maintained with an appropriate hollow tube or airway. Assisted ventilation may be applied directly to the orifice or tube.

Tracheostomy is time consuming and difficult to perform well in emergency situations. It is best undertaken as a formal surgical procedure under optimum conditions. Jet ventilation is preferred to cricothyrotomy when the patient is less than 12 years of age.

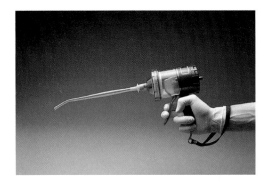

Hand operated pump

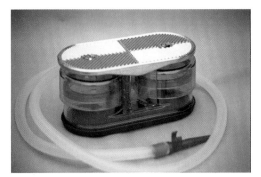

Foot pump

Airway support and ventilation devices

Hygiene considerations
Because of concerns about transmissible viral or bacterial infections, demand has increased for airway adjuncts that prevent direct patient and rescuer contact. This subject is considered further in Chapter 18.

Resuscitation airways may be used to ensure airway patency or isolation, to provide a port for positive pressure ventilation, and to facilitate oxygen enrichment

Barrier or shield devices
These consist of a plastic sheet with a central airway that incorporate a one-way patient valve or filter. Although these devices are compact and inexpensive, they generally do not seal effectively nor maintain airway patency, and may present a high inspiratory resistance, especially when wet. Using an anaesthetic style disposable filter heat and moisture exchanger device on the airway devices described below affords additional protection to patient and rescuer and prevents contamination of self-inflating bags and other equipment.

Tongue support
The oral Guedel airway improves airway patency but requires supplementary jaw support. A short airway will fail to support the tongue; a long airway may stimulate the epiglottis or larynx and induce vomiting or laryngospasm in lightly unconscious patients. Soft nasopharyngeal tubes are better tolerated but may cause nasopharyngeal bleeding, and they require some skill to insert. These simple airways do not protrude from the face and are therefore suitable for use in combination with mask ventilation.

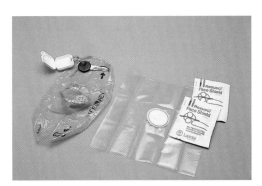

Life key and face shield

Ventilation masks
The use of a ventilation mask during expired air resuscitation, especially when it has a non-rebreathing valve or filter, offers the rescuer protection against direct patient contact. The rescuer seals the mask on the patient's face using a firm

two-handed grip and blows through the mask while lifting the patient's jaw. Transparent masks with well-fitting, air-filled cuffs provide an effective seal on the patient's face and may incorporate valves through which the rescuer can conduct mouth-to-mask ventilation. Detachable valves are preferred, which leave a mask orifice of a standard size into which a self-inflating bag mount (outside diameter 22 mm, inside diameter 15 mm) may be fitted. These enable rapid conversion to bag-valve-mask ventilation.

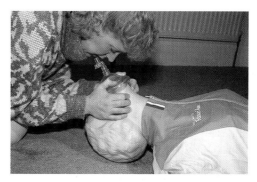

Mouth-to-mask ventilation

Tidal volumes of 700-1000 ml are currently recommended for expired air ventilation by mouth or mask in the absence of supplementary oxygen. Given the difficulty experienced by most rescuers in achieving adequate tidal volumes by mouth or mask ventilation, such guidelines may be difficult to achieve in practice. If the casualty's lips are opposed, only limited air flow may be possible through the nose, and obstructed expiration may be unrecognised in some patients. The insertion of oral or nasal airways is, therefore, advisable when using mask ventilation. Rescuers risk injury when performing mouth-to-mask ventilation in moving vehicles.

Some rescue masks incorporate an inlet port for supplementary oxygen, although in an emergency an oxygen delivery tube can be introduced under the mask cuff or clenched in the rescuer's mouth.

Bag-valve devices
Self-refilling manual resuscitation bags are available that attach to a mask and facilitate bag-valve-mask (BVM) ventilation with air and supplementary oxygen. They are capable of delivering tidal volumes in excess of 800 ml; these volumes are now considered to be excessive, difficult to deliver, and liable to distend the stomach with air. Tidal volumes of 500 ml will suffice if supplementary oxygen in excess of 40% is provided, and smaller devices have been marketed accordingly. Oxygen supplementation through a simple side port on the bag or mask will provide only 35-50% inspired concentration. The addition of oxygen via an oxygen reservoir bag at a flow rate of 8-12 l/min will ensure inspired oxygen levels of 80-95%.

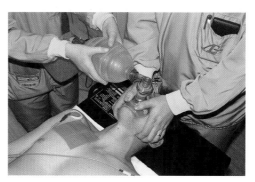

Bag-valve-mask ventilation

For inexperienced rescuers BVM ventilation is difficult because of the need to apply the mask securely while lifting the jaw and squeezing the bag. A firm two-handed grip on the mask may be preferred, with an additional rescuer squeezing the bag. Effective volumes may be more easily achieved by mouth-to-mask than by mouth-to-mouth or bag-valve-mask ventilation

Airway isolation

Tracheal intubation with a cuffed tube, "the definitive airway," is the gold standard for airway protection, allowing positive pressure ventilation of the lungs without gaseous inflation of the stomach, gastric regurgitation, and pulmonary soiling. However, the technique is not easy to perform, requires additional equipment and considerable experience, and is only tolerated at deep levels of unconsciousness. In emergency situations the risk of laryngospasm, regurgitation, vomiting, and misplaced intubation is ever present.

Oropharyngeal, pharyngotracheal, and oesophageal "supraglottic" airways
These devices maintain oral and pharyngolaryngeal patency without jaw support and provide a port for expired air and bag-valve ventilation. The devices have one or two inflatable cuffs that can be inflated in the pharynx and upper oesophagus, permitting positive pressure ventilation and oesophageal isolation, respectively, thereby facilitating their use in anaesthesia and resuscitation for both spontaneous and controlled ventilation. Examples include the pharyngotracheal lumen airway and the Combi-tube.

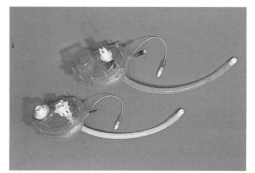

Oesophageal obturators. Top: Esophageal Obturator Airway; lower: Esophageal Gastric Tube Airway

Laryngeal mask airway

This innovative airway adjunct has revolutionised anaesthetic and resuscitation practice. The curved tube, terminating in a spoon-shaped rubber mask with an inflatable rim, is passed blindly into the hypopharynx to isolate and seal the laryngeal inlet. The trachea is thus protected against aspiration from sources both above and below the larynx. Several mask sizes are available to fit patients ranging from babies to large adults. Patients seem to tolerate a laryngeal mask airway (LMA) at a level of consciousness somewhere between that required for an oral airway and a tracheal intubation.

Developments of this device included the flexible reinforced LMA (for head and neck surgery) and the intubating laryngeal mask, which allows the blind passage of a separate soft-tipped, flexible reinforced tracheal tube through the LMA lumen.

Whether the LMA is safe for use with a "full stomach" has been of concern, but its increasing popularity in emergencies by personnel unskilled in tracheal intubation is encouraging. One multicentre trial recorded an incidence of aspiration of only 1.5%. Although competence in LMA insertion can be acquired with minimal training, the high cost of single use versions may preclude its wider acceptance by paramedic and hospital resuscitation services.

Tracheal intubation

This technique entails flexing the patient's neck and extending the head at the atlanto-occipital junction. A laryngoscope is used to expose the epiglottis by lifting the jaw and base of the tongue forward, and the larynx is seen. A curved tube is inserted into the trachea through the vocal cords. Inflation of the tracheal cuff isolates the airway and enables ventilation to be performed safely. The potential risks of the technique include stimulating laryngospasm and vomiting in a semiconscious patient, trauma to the mouth and larynx, unilateral bronchial intubation, unrecognised intubation of the oesophagus, and injury to an unstable cervical spine. If initial attempts at tracheal intubation are not successful within 30 seconds the patient should be reventilated with oxygen and repeat laryngoscopy should be undertaken with careful attention to orolaryngeal alignment. For difficult intubations the careful use of a flexible stylet, its tip kept strictly within the tracheal tube, may help curve and stiffen the tube before intubation. Alternatively, the pre-passage of a long, thin flexible gum-elastic bougie between the cords during laryngoscopy acts as a guide down which to "railroad" the tube into the larynx. Techniques for tracheal intubation that avoid formal laryngoscopy have been advocated, such as blind nasal intubation, digital manipulation of the tube in the laryngopharynx, and transillumination with lighted tube stylets. These have limited success even in experienced hands. If one or two further attempts at intubation are unsuccessful the procedure should be abandoned without delay and alternative methods of airway control chosen.

Accidental oesophageal intubation or tracheal tube dislodgement after initial successful intubation may pass undetected in clothed, restless patients intubated in dark or restricted conditions, or during long transits. The incidence of incorrect intubation varies with experience but some publications report rates of oesophageal intubation by paramedic and emergency medical technicians as high as 17-50%. Simple clinical observation of a rising chest or precordial, lung, and stomach auscultation may be misleading. Confirmation of correct tracheal placement by other techniques is advised. These include the use of an "oesophageal

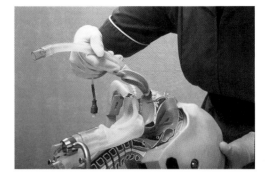

Manikin for practising tracheal intubation

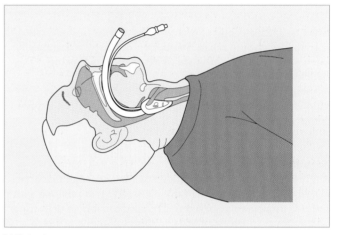

LMA in situ

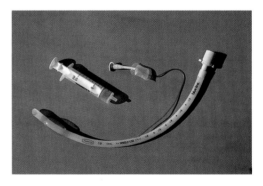

Tracheal tube

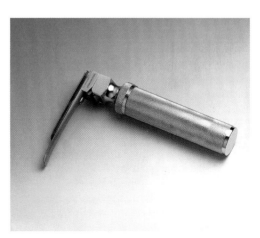

Laryngoscope

detector device," in which unrestricted fast aspiration with a 50 ml syringe or bulb confirms correct tracheal placement, and the use of end-tidal CO_2 monitoring. In the presence of low cardiac output or cardiac arrest when the expired CO_2 may be negligible or non-existent, CO_2 monitoring devices may falsely suggest oesophageal intubation, leading to unnecessary removal of a properly placed tracheal airway.

Supplementary oxygen

Room air contains 21% oxygen, expired air only 16%. In shock, a low cardiac output together with ventilation-perfusion mismatch results in severe hypoxaemia (low arterial oxygen tension). The importance of providing a high oxygen gradient from mouth to vital cells cannot be overemphasised, so oxygen should be added during cardiopulmonary emergencies as soon as it is available. An initial inspired oxygen concentration of 80-100% is desirable. For a self-ventilating patient this is best achieved by a close-fitting oxygen reservoir face mask with a flow rate of 10-12 l/min. For ventilated patients, oxygen at a similar flow rate should be added to the reservoir behind the ventilation bag as explained above. An improvement in the patient's colour is a sign of improved tissue oxygenation.

Portable oximeters with finger or ear probes are increasingly used to measure arterial oxygen saturation, provided an adequate pulsatile blood flow is present; they are useless and misleading in the presence of cardiac arrest. Normal arterial saturation is in excess of 93% compared with a venous saturation of about 75%. Arterial oxygen saturation should be maintained above 90% by combining adequate ventilation with oxygen supplementation. Premature newborns at risk of retrolental fibroplasia and type II chronic respiratory failure patients ("blue bloaters") dependent on a hypoxic drive to breathe are the only rarely encountered patient groups likely to be harmed by prolonged high oxygen therapy.

Physical principles of oxygen therapy devices
Typically these devices are driven from a pressurised oxygen source to which varying amounts of air are added by entrainment. "Entrainment" embraces actions ranging from simple patient activated inspiration to customised Venturi-operated devices.

"Non-reservoir" masks that profess to deliver oxygen at greater than 40% will require high oxygen flows in excess of 10 l/min. By way of example, a 60% "Venturi style" mask requires 15 l/min oxygen flow to generate the required 50:50 oxygen:air mixture to satisfy a peak inspiratory flow of 30 l/min. For oxygen fractions above 60%, masks or resuscitation bags incorporating reservoir bags or large-bore tubes are the only practical answer because these can accumulate oxygen between breaths. Even so, oxygen flows of 12-15 l/min are required to achieve inspired concentrations above 80% in such devices.

> **To maintain the heart and the brain**
> **Give oxygen now and again.**
> **Not now and again,**
> **But NOW, AND AGAIN,**
> **AND AGAIN, AND AGAIN, AND AGAIN.**
> **(Adapted from a well-known limerick)**

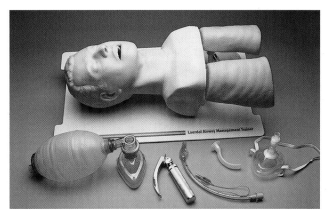

Airway management trainer (Laerdal) allows ventilation of the manikin with a range of airway adjuncts including tracheal intubation

Further reading
- Baskett P, Nolan J, Parr M. Tidal volumes which are perceived to be adequate for resuscitation. *Resuscitation* 1996;31:231-4.
- Brain A. The laryngeal mask—a new concept in airway management. *Br J Anaesthesia* 1983;53:801-5.
- Brain AIJ, Verghese C, Strube PJ. The LMA "ProSeal"—a laryngeal mask with an oesophageal vent. *Br J Anaesthesia* 2000;84:65-74.
- Davies PRF, Tighe SQM, Greenslade GL, Evans GH. Laryngeal mask airway and tracheal tube insertion by unskilled personnel. *Lancet* 1990;336:977-9.
- Gabbott DA, Baskett PJF. Management of the airway and ventilation during resuscitation. *Br J Anaesthesia* 1997;79:159-71.
- International guidelines 2000 for cardiopulmonary resuscitation and emergency cardiovascular care—an international consensus on science. Part 3: adult basic life support. *Resuscitation* 2000;46:29-71.
- International guidelines 2000 for cardiopulmonary resuscitation and emergency cardiovascular care—an international consensus on science. Part 6: Section 1: introduction to ACLS 2000: overview of recommended changes in ACLS from the guidelines 2000 conference. *Resuscitation* 2000; 46:103-7.
- International guidelines 2000 for cardiopulmonary resuscitation and emergency cardiovascular care—an international consensus on science. Part 6: Section 3: adjuncts for oxygenation, ventilation and airway control. *Resuscitation* 2000;46:115-25.
- Oczenski W, Krenn H, Dahaba AA, Binder M, El-Schahawi-Kienzl, Kohout S, et al. Complications following the use of the Combitube, tracheal tube and laryngeal mask airway. *Anaesthesia* 1999;54:1161-5.
- Sellick BA. Cricoid pressure to control regurgitation of stomach contents during induction of anaesthesia. *Lancet* 1961;ii:404-6.
- Stone BJ, Leach AB, Alexander CA. The use of the laryngeal mask airway by nurses during cardiopulmonary resuscitation. Results of a multicentre trial. *Anaesthesia* 1994;49:3-7.
- Tanigawa K, Shigematsu A. Choice of airway devices for 12,020 cases of nontraumatic cardiac arrest in Japan. *Prehosp Emerg Care* 1998;2:96-100.
- Wenzel W, Idris AH, Dorges V, Nolan JP, Parr MJ, Gabrielli A, et al. The respiratory system during resuscitation: a review of the history, risk of infection during assisted ventilation, respiratory mechanics and ventilation strategies for patients with an unprotected airway. *Resuscitation* 2001;49:123-34.

7 Post-resuscitation care

Peter A Oakley, Anthony D Redmond

Full recovery from cardiac arrest is rarely immediate.
The restoration of electrocardiographic complexes and a
palpable pulse mark the start and not the end of a successful
resuscitation attempt. The true endpoint is a fully conscious,
neurologically intact patient with a spontaneous stable cardiac
rhythm and an adequate urine output. The chances of
achieving this are greatly enhanced if the conditions for
successful resuscitation are met.

Once spontaneous cardiac output has been restored, a
senior clinician must consider transferring the patient to an
intensive care area to provide a suitable environment and level
of care to optimise physiological recovery and respond to any
further episodes of cardiac arrest. A decision to keep the
patient on a general ward is rarely appropriate and should only
be made by someone of experience and authority. Implicit in
such a decision is a judgement that the patient's prognosis is so
poor that intensive care will be futile or that, on re-evaluation
of the patient's condition and pre-existing health status, further
resuscitation attempts would be inappropriate. An early
decision to institute palliative care instead of intensive care is
confounded by the difficulty in interpreting the patient's
prognosis on the basis of the immediate post-arrest findings.
If in doubt, it is essential to implement full intensive care and
reconsider the decision later, when the prognosis is more clear.
Before withdrawing active treatment, it is important to seek the
views of the patient's relatives and, if available, the declared
wishes of the patient. However, it is unfair to leave a palliative
care decision entirely to the relatives. Legally, this remains a
medical responsibility, although it is crucial to have the support
of the relatives in making such a decision.

Physiological system support

Post-resuscitation care is based on meticulous physiological
control to optimise recovery. The focus is no longer confined
to airway, breathing, and circulation; other physiological
systems assume particular importance, especially the nervous
system.

Airway and ventilation

In a coronary care unit or similar setting, where immediate
recognition and intervention is at hand, the patient may show
little respiratory compromise after a brief episode of ventricular
fibrillation. Rapid return of an effective cerebral circulation
may restore the gag reflex, protecting the airway from
aspiration. On a general hospital ward, although cardiac arrest
is often witnessed, it may be many minutes before definitive
treatment can be started.

If the time from the onset of cardiac arrest to return of full
consciousness is more than about three minutes, the airway will
be at risk and spontaneous ventilation may be inadequate.
If not already inserted during cardiopulmonary resuscitation
(CPR), a cuffed endotracheal (ET) tube should then be used
to protect the airway, to deliver high-concentration oxygen, to
facilitate control of the ventilation, and to help correct the

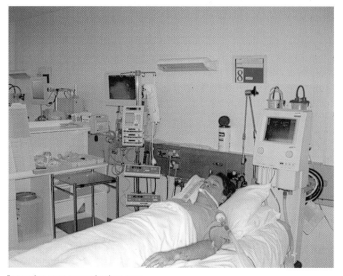

Intensive post-resuscitation care

Successful resuscitation is more likely if:

- Arrest was witnessed
- Underlying arrhythmia was ventricular
  fibrillation
- CPR was started immediately and
  maintained
- Successful cardioversion achieved in
  2-3 minutes and not longer than 8 minutes

Re-establishing perfusion

- Restored cardiac output
- Adequate organ perfusion pressure
- Good oxygenation
- Normal blood glucose

Minimising reperfusion injury

- Hypothermia

---

acidosis. It also provides a route for endobronchial suction of sputum and aspirated material. Depending on the patient's level of consciousness, anaesthesia or sedation will be required to insert the ET tube and to allow it to be tolerated by the patient. This should be administered by an experienced clinician to avoid further cardiovascular compromise and hypoxia. Once an ET tube is in place, it should only be removed after stopping any sedative drugs and checking that the airway reflexes and ventilation have returned to normal.

While manual ventilation with a self-inflating bag is acceptable in the first instance, better control of the pCO_2 is achieved with a mechanical ventilator. The ventilator settings should be adjusted according to frequent blood gas analyses to ensure that the pCO_2 is low enough to help compensate for any severe metabolic acidosis and to avoid cerebral vasodilatation if brain swelling is present; it should not be so low as to cause cerebral vasoconstriction and further brain ischaemia. "Low normal" values of 4.5-5.0 kPa are generally appropriate. It is important not to rely on end-tidal CO_2 values as an estimate of pCO_2. They are inaccurate in the face of a compromised circulation or ventilation-perfusion abnormalities within the lung.

Early attempts at mouth-to-mouth or bag-valve-mask ventilation may have introduced air into the stomach. An initially misplaced tracheal tube will do the same. Gastric distension provokes vomiting, is uncomfortable, and impairs ventilation. It is important to decompress the stomach with a nasogastric tube.

A chest radiograph is an essential early adjunct to post-resuscitation care. It may show evidence of pulmonary oedema or aspiration and allows the position of the ET tube and central venous line to be checked. It may also show mechanical complications of CPR, such as a pneumothorax or rib fractures. Remember too that vigorous CPR can cause an anterior flail segment leading to severe pain and impaired ventilatory capacity.

Circulation

The haemodynamics of the period after cardiac arrest are complex and further arrhythmias are likely. Continuous electrocardiographic monitoring is mandatory and guides therapy for arrhythmias. Thrombolysis may be contraindicated after CPR as the associated physical trauma makes the patient vulnerable to haemorrhage, especially if the arrest has been prolonged. However, if the period of CPR is short, the benefits of thrombolysis may outweigh the risks.

Survivors of cardiac arrest may have acute coronary artery occlusion that is difficult to predict clinically or on electrocardiographic findings. Coronary angiography and angioplasty should be considered in suitable candidates.

Invasive monitoring should be considered in any patient who is intubated or who requires the administration of haemodynamically active drugs after cardiac arrest.

An indwelling arterial catheter is invaluable for monitoring the blood pressure on a beat-to-beat basis, at the same time allowing repeated blood gas estimations to monitor the effects of ventilation and identify disturbances in the electrolytes and acid-base balance.

A pulmonary artery catheter, transoesophageal Döppler monitor, or pulse contour cardiac output (PiCCO) monitor allows haemodynamic variables (directly measured or derived by computer algorithms) to be tracked and adjusted by the careful use of fluids, inotropes, vasodilators, or diuretics. The benefits of a pulmonary artery catheter must be weighed against the risks of its placement through the heart, precipitating further arrhythmias. A transoesophageal Döppler

---

Immediately after restoration of a cardiac rhythm complete the following checklist

- Ensure that the ET tube is correctly placed in the trachea, using direct laryngoscopy or end-tidal CO_2 monitoring
- Ensure that the patient is being adequately ventilated with 100% oxygen. Listen with a stethoscope and confirm adequate and equal air entry. If pneumothorax is suspected insert a chest drain
- Measure arterial pH and gases, repeating frequently
- Measure urea, creatinine and electrolytes, including calcium and magnesium
- Measure plasma glucose
- Obtain a chest radiograph.
- Insert a urinary catheter and measure the urinary output
- Insert a nasogastic tube and aspirate the contents of the stomach
- Obtain a 12 lead electrocardiogram
- Measure cardiac enzymes

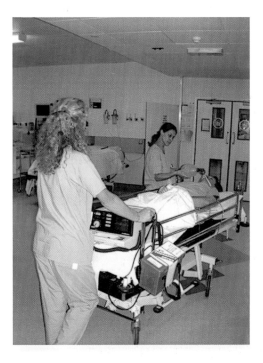

Transfer to the intensive care unit

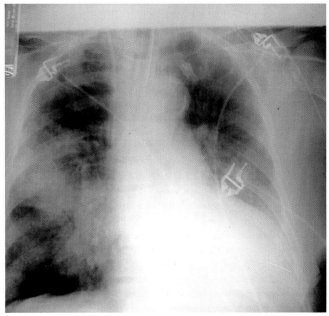

A check chest x ray is essential

monitor, while less accurate, is less invasive and has fewer risks, but can only be used in intubated patients. The PiCCO device requires a central venous catheter and a large-bore arterial cannula to be inserted. It allows estimates of cardiac index, systemic vascular resistance, intrathoracic blood volume, and extravascular lung water to be made.

Transthoracic or transoesophageal echocardiography provides a more detailed snapshot of cardiac function, but is more operator dependent. It allows ventricular wall and valve movements to be visualised, an estimate of ejection fraction to be made, and overall cardiac performance to be judged.

Neurological management

After cardiac arrest, special attention must be paid to ongoing cerebral resuscitation. Although cardiovascular compromise is likely, it is neurological dysfunction that tends to cause most concern.

The brain suffers further harm when its blood flow is restored. Reperfusion injury results from a cascade of events occurring in brain tissue. Intracellular levels of glutamate increase and an excitatory neurotransmitter is released from presynaptic terminals. This activates ion channels, causing calcium to be transported from the extracellular to the intracellular fluid. This, in turn, leads to the accumulation of oxygen free radicals and the activation of degradative enzymes.

Pharmacological interventions, including thiopentone, steroids, and nimodopine, have not be shown to be of benefit in preventing or kerbing reperfusion injury. Recent studies have shown that lowering the body temperature to 32-34°C (mild hypothermia) for 12-24 hours in comatose survivors can improve both survival and neurological outcome. Hypothermia lowers the glutamate level, reducing the production of oxygen free radicals. It may also decrease intracranial pressure (ICP) but is associated with a lower cardiac index, higher systemic vascular resistance, and hyperglycaemia. Temperatures below 32°C should be avoided because they are associated with a high risk of arrhythmias. Cooling can be conveniently achieved by the use of an external device consisting of a mattress with a cover, delivering cold air over the entire body surface (TheraKool, Kinetic Concepts, Wareham, United Kingdom), supplemented by the use of ice packs if it is proving difficult to achieve the target temperature.

Other secondary insults after resuscitation include seizures and intracranial hypertension. If mechanical ventilation and muscle relaxants are being used, "clinical" fits may not be recognised. Remember that subclinical seizures may also occur and will only be evident using EEG techniques.

Cerebral perfusion depends on an adequate mean arterial pressure (MAP). Although monitoring ICP can inform the clinician about the cerebral perfusion pressure (CPP = MAP − ICP), no evidence has been found to show that such monitoring is beneficial in this situation. If the ICP is raised to 20 mm Hg, elevating the MAP to 90 mm Hg would provide a "neurosurgical" target CPP of 70 mm Hg, but driving the heart too hard may threaten an already compromised myocardium. Nevertheless, it is wise to choose an MAP target of at least 80 mm Hg (and ideally 90 mm Hg) if raised ICP is strongly suspected. Careful cardiovascular monitoring may help to achieve and maintain what can be a very delicate balance. The potential benefits of vasodilator drugs that reduce cardiac afterload must be balanced against their potential threat to CPP.

Judging the prognosis in patients who remain comatose after cardiac arrest is fraught with problems. Although fixed dilated pupils are worrying, they are not reliable as an indicator of outcome. Hypercarbia, atropine, and adrenaline

> When the heart stops the brain may be damaged by the initial ischaemia and by the reduced cerebral perfusion that is inevitable, even with high quality CPR. When cerebral blood flow ceases the electroencephalogram (EEG) becomes flat within 10 seconds and cerebral glucose is used up within one minute. Microthrombi and sludging occur in the myriad of tiny cerebral vessels. While neuronal activity may continue for up to one hour, a good neurological outcome is unlikely after more than three minutes of arrested circulation at normal ambient temperatures

> Grand mal fits are common and do not by themselves imply a poor prognosis. Treatment with phenytoin should be instituted, with careful haemodynamic monitoring. Focal fits and myoclonic jerks are also common and may not respond to phenytoin. Drugs, such as sodium valproate and clonazepam, should be considered for focal fits and myoclonic jerks, respectively. Myoclonic jerks were previously considered to indicate a dismal prognosis but many patients make a good recovery, especially young patients in whom the cause of cardiac arrest was respiratory rather than cardiovascular (for example, acute severe asthma)

> In patients who remain unconscious without sedation 72 hours after a cardiac arrest, the absense of cortical somato-sensory evoked potentials (SSEPs) has been claimed to be a reliable indicator of poor outcome. Others consider it necessary to wait for a week before SSEPs can predict poor outcome with certainty. Such delays are frustrating when a good outcome seems unlikely. In the absence of other reasons to institute palliative care, full care should be continued for up to a week before making a final evaluation, especially in otherwise fit patients whose cardiac arrest had been caused by hypoxia rather than by a primary cardiac arrhythmia

(epinephrine) may all cause this sign in the immediate post-arrest phase.

Early indicators of poor outcome have proved elusive, hampering palliative care decisions. The absence of motor function at 72 hours has been used as a predictor, but may be affected by residual sedative drugs in the circulation. Adjunct investigations, such as computerised tomography scan, magnetic resonance imaging, and EEG, may be helpful. However, it may be several days before a CT scan will show cerebral infarction and the EEG may be affected by residual sedation. MRI is useful in the diagnosis of global ischaemic encephalopathy. Biochemical markers such as neutron-specific enolase in blood and cerebrospinal fluid may offer supportive evidence of severe brain injury.

Metabolic problems

Meticulous control of pH and electrolyte balance is an essential part of post-arrest management. Bicarbonate, with its well-recognised complications (shift of the oxygen dissociation curve to the left, sodium and osmolar load, paradoxical intracellular acidosis, and hypokalaemia), should be avoided if possible. If used, it should be carefully titrated in small doses, using repeated arterial sampling to monitor its effects. Hypokalaemia may have precipitated the original cardiac arrest, particularly in elderly patients taking digoxin and diuretics. Potassium may be administered by a central line in doses of up to 40 mmol in an hour.

A low serum magnesium concentration can also cause arrhythmias. As it has few side effects, magnesium can be safely administered to patients with frequent ectopics or atrial fibrillation without waiting for laboratory confirmation of hypomagnesaemia. Even when the level is normal, the administration of magnesium may suppress arrhythmias.

A urinary catheter and graduated collection bottle are necessary to monitor urine output. An adequate cardiac output and blood pressure should produce 40-50 ml of urine every hour.

Conclusion

A commitment to treat cardiac arrest is a commitment to critical care after resuscitation. The patient who survives should generally be managed in an intensive care unit and is likely to need at least a short period of mechanical ventilation. If the conscious level does not return rapidly to normal, induced hypothermia should be considered.

Predicting longer term neurological outcome in the immediate post-arrest period is fraught with difficulties. The initial clinical signs are not reliable indicators. The duration of the arrest and the duration and degree of post-arrest coma have some predictive value but can be misleading. Although not valid immediately after the arrest, electrophysiological tests, especially SSEPs, are valuable adjuncts to support a clinical judgement of very poor neurological recovery.

Unless an informed, senior opinion has been sought, received, and agreed, the decision to resuscitate must always be followed by full post-resuscitation care.

Blood glucose may rise as a stress response, particularly if there has been a serious cerebral insult, and this may be exacerbated by adrenaline (epinephrine) or underlying diabetes. Blood glucose levels should be kept within the normal range to avoid the harmful effects of both hyperglycaemia (increase in cerebral metabolism) and hypoglycaemia (loss of the brain's major energy source)

A prolonged period of cardiac arrest or a persistently low cardiac output after restoration of a spontaneous circulation may precipitate acute renal failure, especially in the face of pre-existing renal impairment. It may be necessary to consider haemofiltration for urgent correction of intractable acidosis, fluid overload, or severe hyperkalaemia, and to manage established renal failure in the medium term. In renal failure after cardiac arrest, remember to adjust the doses of renally excreted drugs such as digoxin to avoid toxicity

---

Further reading

- Bernard SA, Gray TW, Buist MD, Jones BM, Silvester W, Gutteridge G, et al. Treatment of comatose survivors of out-of-hospital cardiac arrest with induced hypothermia. *N Eng J Med* 2002;346:557-63.
- Inamasu J, Ichikizaki K. Mild hypothermia in neurological emergency: an update. *Ann Emerg Med* 2002;40:220-30.
- Jorgensen EO, Holm S. The course of circulatory and cerebral recovery after circulatory arrest: influence of pre-arrest, arrest and post-arrest factors. *Resuscitation* 1999;42:173-82.
- Morris HR, Howard RS, Brown P. Early myoclonic status and outcome after cardiorespiratory arrest. *J Neurol Neurosurg Psychiatry* 1998;64:267-8.
- Premachandran S, Redmond AD, Liddle R, Jones JM. Cardiopulmonary arrest in general wards: a retrospective study of referral patterns to an intensive care facility and their influence on outcome. *J Accid Emerg Med* 1997;14:26-9.
- Robertson CE. *Cardiac arrest and cardiopulmonary resuscitation in adults. Cambridge textbook of accident and emergency medicine.* Cambridge: Cambridge University Press, 1997, pp. 62-80.
- The Hypothermia After Cardiac Arrest Study Group. Mild therapeutic hypothermia to improve the neurologic outcome after cardiac arrest. *N Eng J Med* 2002;346:549-56.
- Zandbergen EGJ, de Haan RJ, Stoutenbeek CP, Koelman JHTM, Hijdra A. Systematic review of early prediction of poor outcome in anoxic-ischaemic coma. *Lancet* 1998;352:1808-12.

8 Resuscitation in pregnancy

Stephen Morris, Mark Stacey

Cardiac arrest occurs only about once in every 30 000 late pregnancies, but survival from such an event is exceptional. Most deaths are due to acute causes, with many mothers receiving some form of resuscitation. However, the number of indirect deaths—that is, deaths from medical conditions exacerbated by pregnancy—is greater than from conditions that arise from pregnancy itself. The use of national guidelines can decrease mortality, an example being the reduction in the number of deaths due to pulmonary embolus and sepsis after caesarean section. In order to try and reduce mortality from amniotic fluid embolism, a national database for suspected cases has been established.

Factors peculiar to pregnancy that weigh the balance against survival include anatomical changes that make it difficult to maintain a clear airway and perform intubation, pathological changes such as laryngeal oedema, physiological factors such as increased oxygen consumption, and an increased likelihood of pulmonary aspiration. In the third trimester the most important factor is compression of the inferior vena cava and impaired venous return by the gravid uterus when the woman lies supine. These difficulties may be exaggerated by obesity. All staff directly or indirectly concerned with obstetric care need to be trained in resuscitation skills.

A speedy response is essential. Once respiratory or cardiac arrest has been diagnosed the patient must be positioned appropriately and basic life support started immediately. This must be continued while venous access is secured, any obvious causal factors are corrected (for example, hypovolaemia), and the necessary equipment, drugs, and staff are assembled.

Basic life support

Airway
A clear airway must be quickly established with head tilt-jaw thrust or head tilt-chin lift manoeuvres, and then maintained. Suction should be used to aspirate vomit. Badly fitting dentures and other foreign bodies should be removed from the mouth and an airway should be inserted. These procedures should be performed with the patient inclined laterally or supine, with the uterus displaced as described on the next page.

Breathing
In the absence of adequate respiration, intermittent positive pressure ventilation should be started once the airway has been cleared; mouth-to-mouth, mouth-to-nose, or mouth-to-airway ventilation should be carried out until a self-inflating bag and mask are available. Ventilation should then be continued with 100% oxygen using a reservoir bag. Because of the increased risk of regurgitation and pulmonary aspiration of gastric contents in late pregnancy, cricoid pressure (see Chapter 6) should be applied until the airway has been protected by a cuffed tracheal tube.

Ventilation is made more difficult by the increased oxygen requirements and reduced chest compliance that occur in pregnancy, the latter due to rib flaring and splinting of the

---

Physiological changes in late pregnancy relevant to cardiopulmonary resuscitation

Respiratory
- Increased ventilation
- Increased oxygen demand
- Reduced chest compliance
- Reduced functional residual capacity

Cardiovascular
- Incompetent gastroesophageal (cardiac) sphincter
- Increased intragastric pressure
- Increased risk of regurgitation

Specific difficulties in pregnant patients

Airway
Patient inclined laterally for:
- Suction or aspiration
- Removing dentures or foreign bodies
- Inserting airways

Breathing
- Greater oxygen requirement
- Reduced chest compliance
- More difficult to see rise and fall of chest
- More risk of regurgitation and aspiration

Circulation
External chest compression difficult because:
- Ribs flared
- Diaphragm raised
- Patient obese
- Breasts hypertrophied
- Supine position causes inferior vena cava
- Compression by the gravid uterus

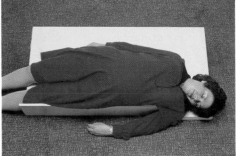

Inclined lateral position using Cardiff wedge

Anatomical features relevant to difficult intubation or ventilation

- Full dentition
- Large breasts
- Oedema or obesity of neck
- Supraglottic oedema
- Flared ribcage
- Raised diaphragm

---

diaphragm by the abdominal contents. Observing the rise and fall of the chest in such patients is also more difficult.

Circulation

Circulatory arrest is diagnosed by the absence of a palpable pulse in a large artery (carotid or femoral). Chest compressions at the standard rate (see Chapter 1) and ratio of 15:2 are given. Chest compression on a pregnant woman is made difficult by flared ribs, raised diaphragm, obesity, and breast hypertrophy. Because the diaphragm is pushed cephalad by the abdominal contents the hand position for chest compressions should similarly be moved up the sternum, although currently no guidelines suggest exactly how far. In the supine position an additional factor is compression of the inferior vena cava by the gravid uterus, which impairs venous return and so reduces cardiac output; all attempts at resuscitation will be futile unless the compression is relieved. This is achieved either by placing the patient in an inclined lateral position by using a wedge or by displacing the uterus manually. Raising the patient's legs will improve venous return.

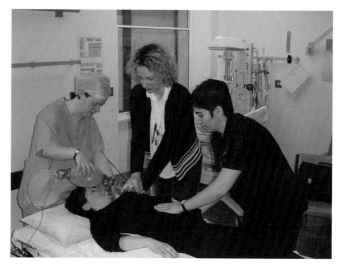

Manual displacement of uterus

Lateral displacement of the uterus

Effective forces for chest compression can be generated with patients inclined at angles of up to 30°, but pregnant women tend to roll into a full lateral position when inclined at angles greater than this, making chest compression difficult. The Cardiff resuscitation wedge is not commercially available, so other techniques need to be used. One technique is the "human wedge," in which the patient is tilted onto a rescuer's knees to provide a stable position for basic life support. Alternatively, the patient can be tilted onto the back of an upturned chair. Purpose-made wedges are available in maternity units, but any available cushion or pillow can be used to wedge the patient into the left inclined position. An assistant should, however, move the uterus further off the inferior vena cava by bimanually lifting it to the left and towards the patient's head.

Advanced life support

Intubation

Tracheal intubation should be carried out as soon as facilities and skill are available. Difficulty in tracheal intubation is more common in pregnant women, and specialised equipment for advanced airway management may be required. A short obese neck and full breasts due to pregnancy may make it difficult to insert the laryngoscope into the mouth. The use of a short handled laryngoscope or one with its blade mounted at more than 90° (polio or adjustable blade) or demounting the blade from the handle during its insertion into the mouth may help.

Mouth-to-mouth or bag and mask ventilation is best undertaken without pillows under the head and with the head and neck fully extended. The position for intubation, however, requires at least one pillow to flex the neck and extend the head. The pillow removed to facilitate initial ventilation must, therefore, be kept at hand for intubation.

In the event of failure to intubate the trachea or ventilate the patient's lungs with a bag and mask, insertion of a laryngeal mask airway (LMA) should be attempted. Cricoid pressure must be temporarily removed in order to place the LMA successfully. Once the LMA is in place, cricoid pressure should be reapplied.

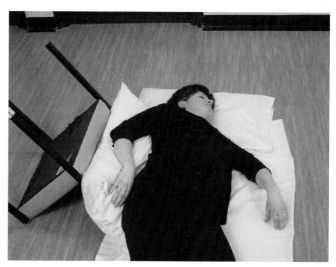

Alternative method for lateral position

Defibrillation and drugs

Defibrillation and drug administration is in accordance with advanced life support recommendations. On a practical note,

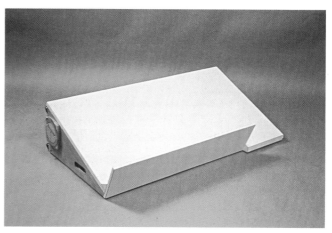

Cardiff wedge

it is difficult to apply an apical defibrillator paddle with the patient inclined laterally, and great care must be taken to ensure that the dependant breast does not come into contact with the hand holding the paddle. This problem is avoided if adhesive electrodes are used.

Increasingly, magnesium sulphate is used for the treatment and prevention of eclampsia. If a high serum magnesium concentration has contributed to the cardiac arrest, consider giving calcium chloride. Tachyarrhythmias due to toxicity by the anaesthetic agent bupivacaine are probably best treated by electrical cardioversion or with bretylium rather than lidocaine (lignocaine).

Caesarean section

This is not merely a last ditch attempt to save the life of the fetus, but it plays an important part in the resuscitation of the mother. Many successful resuscitations have occurred after prompt surgical intervention. The probable mechanism for the favourable outcome is that occlusion of the inferior vena cava is relieved completely by emptying the uterus, whereas it is only partially relieved by manual uterine displacement or an inclined position. Delivery also improves thoracic compliance, which will improve the efficacy of chest compressions and the ability to ventilate the lungs.

After cardiac arrest, non-pregnant adults suffer irreversible brain damage from anoxia within three to four minutes, but pregnant women become hypoxic more quickly. Although evidence shows that the fetus can tolerate prolonged periods of hypoxia, the outlook for the neonate is optimised by immediate caesarean section.

If maternal cardiac arrest occurs in the labour ward, operating theatre, or accident and emergency department, and basic and advanced life support are not successful within five minutes, the uterus should be emptied by surgical intervention. Given the time taken to prepare theatre packs, this procedure is probably best carried out with just a scalpel. Time will pass very quickly in such a high-pressure situation, and it is advisable to practise this scenario, particularly in the accident and emergency department. Cardiopulmonary resuscitation must be continued throughout the operation and afterwards because this improves the prognosis for mother and child. If necessary, transabdominal open cardiac massage can be performed. After successful delivery both mother and infant should be transferred to their appropriate intensive care units as soon as clinical conditions permit. The key factor for successful resuscitation in late pregnancy is that all midwifery, nursing, and medical staff concerned with obstetric care should be trained in cardiopulmonary resuscitation.

Retention of cardiopulmonary resuscitation skills is poor, particularly in midwives and obstetricians who have little opportunity to practise them. Regular short periods of practice on a manikin are therefore essential.

Members of the public and the ambulance service should be aware of the additional problems associated with resuscitation in late pregnancy. The training of ambulance staff is of particular importance as paramedics are likely to be the primary responders to community obstetric emergency calls.

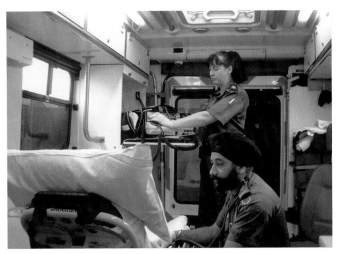

Paramedics are often the primary responders to obstetric emergency calls, and so awareness of problems associated with resuscitation in late pregnancy is important

> The timing of caesarean section and the speed with which surgical delivery is carried out is critical in determining the outcome for mother and fetus. Most of the children and mothers who survive emergency caesarean deliveries are delivered within five minutes of maternal cardiac arrest

Further reading

- Department of Health. *Report on Confidential enquiry into maternal deaths in the United Kingdom 1997–1999*. London: HMSO, 2001.
- European Resuscitation Council. Part 8: Advanced challenges in resuscitation. Section 3: Special challenges in ECC. 3F: Cardiac arrest associated with pregnancy. *Resuscitation* 2000;46:293-5.
- Goodwin AP, Pearce AJ. The human wedge: a manoeuvre to relieve aortocaval compression in resuscitation during late pregnancy. *Anaesthesia* 1992;47:433-4.
- Page-Rodriguez A, Gonzalez-Sanchez JA. Perimortem cesarean section of twin pregnancy: case report and review of the literature. *Acad Emerg Med* 1999;6:1072-4.
- Whitten M, Irvine LM. Postmortem and perimortem cesarean section: what are the indications? *J R Soc Med* 2000;93:6-9.

9 Resuscitation at birth

Anthony D Milner

The first priority for all those responsible for the care of babies at birth must be to ensure that adequate resuscitation facilities are available. Sadly, some babies have irreversible brain damage by the time of delivery, but it is unacceptable that any damage should occur after delivery due to inadequate equipment or insufficiently trained staff. For this reason, there should always be at least two healthcare professionals at all deliveries—one who is primarily responsible for the care of the mother, and the other, who must be trained in basic neonatal resuscitation, to look after the baby.

All babies known to be at increased risk should be delivered in a unit with full respiratory support facilities and must always be attended by a doctor who is skilled in resuscitation and solely responsible for the care of that baby. Whenever possible, there should also be a trained assistant who can provide additional help if necessary. Babies at increased risk make up about a quarter of all deliveries and about two thirds of those requiring resuscitation; the remaining one third are babies born after a normal uneventful labour who have no apparent risk factors. Staff on labour wards must, therefore, always be prepared to provide adequate resuscitation until further help can be obtained.

Equipment

The padded platform on which the baby is resuscitated can either be flat or have a head-down tilt. It can be wall mounted or kept on a trolley, provided that one is available for each delivery area. It is essential that there should be an overhead heater with an output of 300-500 Watts mounted about 1 m above the platform. This must have a manual control because servo systems are slow to set up and likely to malfunction when the baby's skin is wet. These heaters are essential, as even in environments of 20-24 °C the core temperature of an asphyxiated wet baby can drop by 5 °C in as many minutes.

Facilities must be available for facemask and tracheal tube resuscitation. The laryngeal mask airway is also potentially useful. The use of oxygen versus air during resuscitation at birth is controversial because high concentrations of oxygen may be toxic in some circumstances. The current international recommendation is that 100% oxygen should be used initially if it is available. As the latest generation of resuscitation systems have air and oxygen mixing facilities it will usually be possible to reduce the inspired oxygen fraction to a lower level once the initial phase of resuscitation is over. Additional equipment needed includes an overhead light, a clock with a second hand, suction equipment, stethoscope, an electrocardiogram (ECG) monitor, and an oxygen saturation monitor.

Procedure at delivery

It is common practice during labour to aspirate the pharynx with a catheter as soon as the face appears. But this is almost always unnecessary unless the amniotic fluid is stained with meconium or blood. Aggressive pharyngeal suction can delay the onset of spontaneous respiration for a considerable time. Once the baby is delivered the attendant should wipe any

---

High-risk deliveries

Delivery
- Fetal distress
- Reduced fetal movement
- Abnormal presentation
- Prolapsed cord
- Antepartum haemorrhage
- Meconium staining of liquor
- High forceps
- Ventouse
- Caesarean section under general anaesthetic

Maternal
- Severe pregnancy-induced hypertension
- Heavy sedation
- Drug addiction
- Diabetes mellitus
- Chronic illness

Fetal
- Multiple pregnancy
- Pre-term ($< 34/52$)
- Post-term ($> 42/52$)
- Small for dates
- Rhesus isoimmunisation
- Hydramnios and oligohydramnios
- Abnormal baby

Resuscitation equipment
- Padded shelf or resuscitation trolley
- Overhead heater
- Overhead light
- Oxygen and air supply
- Clock
- Stethoscope
- Airway pressure manometer and pressure relief valve
- Facemask
- Oropharyngeal airways 00, +0
- Resuscitation system (facemask, T-piece, bag and mask)
- Suction catheters (sized 5, 8, 10 gauge)
- Mechanical and/or manual suction with double trap
- Two laryngoscopes with spare blades
- Tracheal tubes 2, 2.5, 3, 3.5, and 4 mm, introducer
- Laryngeal masks
- Umbilical vein catheterisation set
- 2, 10, and 20 ml syringes with needles
- Intraosseous needle
- ECG and transcutaneous oxygen saturation monitor
- Note: capnometers are a strongly recommended optional extra

excess fluid off the baby with a warm towel to reduce evaporative heat loss, while examining the child for major external congenital abnormalities such as spina bifida and severe microcephaly. Most babies will start breathing during this period as the median time until the onset of spontaneous respiration is only 10 seconds. They can then be handed to their parents. If necessary, the baby can be encouraged to breathe by skin stimulation—for example, flicking the baby's feet; those not responding must be transferred immediately to the resuscitation area.

Resuscitation procedure

Once it is recognised that the newborn baby is failing to breathe spontaneously and adequately, the procedures standardised in the *International Resuscitation Guidelines* published in 2000 should be followed. These guidelines acknowledge that few resuscitation interventions have been subjected to randomised controlled trials. However, there have been a number of small physiological studies on the effects of these interventions.

Check first for respiratory efforts and listen and feel for air movement. If respiratory movements are present, even if they are vigorous, but there is no tidal exchange, then the airway is obstructed. This can usually be overcome by placing the head in a neutral position (which may require a small roll of cloth under the shoulders) and gently lifting the chin. An oropharyngeal airway may occasionally be required, particularly if the baby has congenital upper airway obstruction, such as choanal atresia.

If respiratory efforts are feeble or totally absent, count the heart rate for 10-15 seconds with a stethoscope over the praecordium. If the heart rate is higher than 80 beats/min it is sufficient to repeat skin stimulation, but if this fails to improve respiration then proceed to facemask resuscitation.

Facemask resuscitation

Only facemasks with a soft continuous ring provide an adequate seal. Most standard devices for manual resuscitation of the neonate fail to produce adequate tidal exchange when the pressure-limiting device is unimpeded. Thus, a satisfactory outcome almost always depends on the inflation pressure stimulating the baby to make spontaneous inspiratory efforts (Head's paradoxical reflex). Tidal exchange can be increased by using a 500 ml rather than a 250 ml reservoir, which allows inflation pressure to be maintained for up to one second.

More satisfactory tidal exchange can be achieved with a T-piece system. In this system, a continuous flow of air and oxygen is led directly into the facemask at 4-6 l/min; the lungs are inflated by intermittently occluding the outlet from the mask. It is essential to incorporate a pressure valve into the fresh gas tubing so that the pressure cannot exceed 30 cmH$_2$O. The baby's lungs are inflated at a rate of about 30/min, allowing one second for each part of the cycle. Listen to the baby's chest after 5-10 inflations to check for bilateral air entry and a satisfactory heart rate. If the heart rate falls below 80 beats/min proceed immediately to tracheal intubation.

Tracheal intubation

Most operators find a straight-bladed laryngoscope preferable for performing neonatal intubation. This is held in the left hand with the baby's neck gently extended, if necessary by the assistant. The laryngoscope is passed to the right of the tongue, ensuring that it is swept to the left of the blade, which is advanced until the epiglottis comes into view. The tip of the

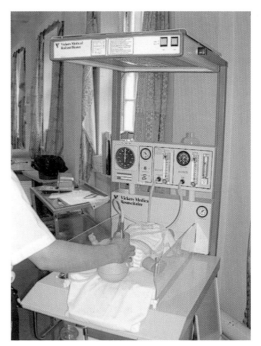

Neonatal resuscitation trolley

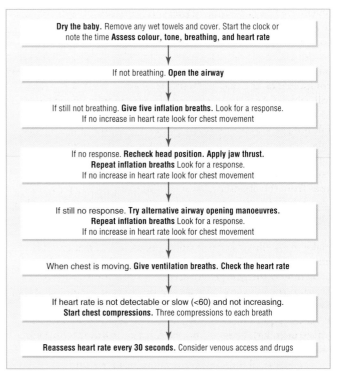

Algorithm for newborn life support. Adapted from *Newborn Life Support Manual*, London: Resuscitation Council (UK)

blade can then be positioned either proximal to or just under the epiglottis so that the cords are brought into view. Gentle backward pressure over the larynx may be needed at this stage. As the upper airway tends to be filled with fluid it may have to be cleared with the suction catheter held in the right hand.

Once the cords are visible, pass the tracheal tube with the right hand and remove the laryngoscope blade, taking care that this does not displace the tube out of the larynx. Most people find it necessary to use an introducer to stiffen straight tracheal tubes. It is then essential to ensure that the tip of the introducer does not protrude, to avoid tracheal and mediastinal perforation. If intubation proves difficult, because the anatomy of the upper airway is abnormal or because of a lack of adequately trained personnel, then a laryngeal mask may be inserted.

Attach the tracheal tube either to a T-piece system incorporating a 30-40 cmH$_2$O blow-off valve (see above) or to a neonatal manual resuscitation device. If a T-piece is used, maintain the initial inflation pressure for two to three seconds. This will help lung expansion. The baby can subsequently be ventilated at a rate of 30/min, allowing about one second for each inflation.

Inspect the chest during the first few inflations, looking for evidence of chest wall movement, and confirm by auscultation that gas is entering both lungs. If no air is entering the lungs then the most likely cause is that the tip of the tracheal tube is lying in the oesophagus. If this is suspected, remove the tube immediately and oxygenate with a mask system. If auscultation shows that gas is entering one lung only, usually the right, withdraw the tube by 1 cm while listening over the lungs. If this leads to improvement, the tip of the tracheal tube was lying in the main bronchus. If no improvement is seen then the possible causes include pneumothorax, diaphragmatic hernia, or pleural effusion.

Severe bradycardia

If the heart rate falls below 60 beats/min, chest compression must be started by pressing with the tips of two fingers over sternum at a point that is one finger's breadth below an imaginary line joining the nipples. If there are two rescuers it is preferable for one to encircle the chest with the hands and compress the same point with the thumbs, while the other carries out ventilation. The chest should be compressed by about one third of its diameter. Give one inflation for every three chest compressions at a rate of about 120 "events" per minute. This will achieve about 90 compressions each minute. Those babies who fail to respond require 10 mcg/kg (0.1 ml/kg of 1/10 000 solution) of adrenaline (epinephrine) given down the tracheal tube. If no improvement is seen within 10-15 seconds the umbilical vein should be catheterised with a 5 French gauge catheter. This is best achieved by transecting the cord 2-3 cm away from the abdominal skin and inserting a catheter until blood flows freely up the catheter. The same dose of adrenaline (epinephrine) can then be given directly into the circulation.

Although evidence shows that sodium bicarbonate can make intracellular acidosis worse, its use can often lead to improvement, and the current recommendation is that the baby should then be given 1-2 mmol/kg of body weight over two to three minutes. This should be given as 2-4 ml/kg of 4.2% solution. Those who fail to respond, or who are in asystole, require further doses of adrenaline (epinephrine) (10-30 mcg/kg). This can be given either intravenously or injected down the tracheal tube.

It is reasonable to continue with alternate doses of adrenaline (epinephrine) and sodium bicarbonate for 20 minutes, even in those who are born in apparent asystole,

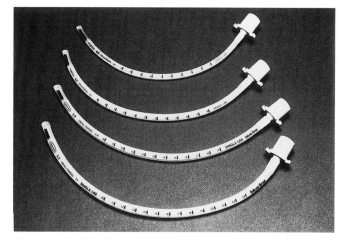

Neonatal tracheal intubation equipment

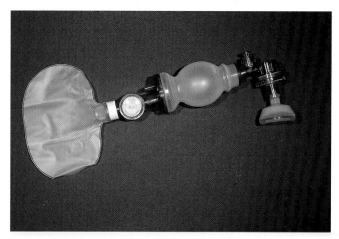

Bag mask for neonatal resuscitation

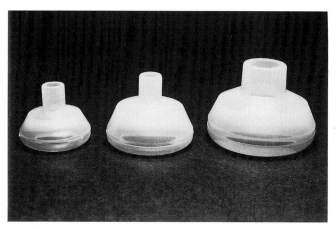

Paediatric face masks.

provided that a fetal heart beat was noted at some time within 15 minutes of delivery. Resuscitation efforts should not be continued beyond 20 minutes unless the baby is making at least intermittent respiratory efforts.

Naloxone therapy

Intravenous or intramuscular naloxone (100 mcg/kg) should be given to all babies who become pink and have an obviously satisfactory circulation after positive pressure ventilation but fail to start spontaneous respiratory efforts. Often the mothers have a history of recent opiate sedation. Alternatively, naloxone can be given down the tracheal tube. If naloxone is effective then an additional 200 micrograms/kg may be given intramuscularly to prevent relapse. Naloxone must not be given to infants of mothers addicted to opiates because this will provoke severe withdrawal symptoms.

Meconium aspiration

A recent large, multicentre, randomised trial has shown that vigorous babies born through meconium should be treated conservatively. The advice for babies with central nervous system depression and thick meconium staining of the liquor remains—that direct laryngoscopy should be carried out immediately after birth. If this shows meconium in the pharynx and trachea, the baby should be intubated immediately and suction applied directly to the tracheal tube, which should then be withdrawn. Provided the baby's heart rate remains above 60 beats/min this procedure can be repeated until meconium is no longer recovered.

Hypovolaemia

Acute blood loss from the baby during delivery may complicate resuscitation. It is not always clear that the baby has bled, so it is important to consider this possibility in any baby who remains pale with rapid small-volume pulses after adequate gas exchange has been achieved. Most babies respond well to a bolus (20-25 ml/kg) of an isotonic saline solution. It is rarely necessary to provide the baby with blood in the labour suite.

Pre-term babies

Babies with a gestation of more than 32 weeks do not differ from full-term babies in their requirement for resuscitation. At less than this gestation they may have a lower morbidity and mortality if a more active intervention policy is adopted. However, no evidence has been found to show that a rigid policy of routine intubation for all babies with a gestation of less than 28 or 30 weeks leads to an improved outcome. Indeed, unless the operator is extremely skilful, this intervention may produce hypoxia in a previously lively pink baby and predispose to intraventricular haemorrhage. A reasonable compromise is to start facemask resuscitation after 15-30 seconds, unless the baby has entirely adequate respiratory efforts, and proceed to intubation if the baby has not achieved satisfactory respiratory efforts by 30-60 seconds. This policy may need to be modified for the delivery of prophylactic surfactant therapy, or if the neonatal unit is a considerable distance from the labour suite.

Evidence is increasing to show that the pre-term baby is at greatest risk from overinflation of the lungs immediately after birth, and inflation volumes as little as 8 ml/kg may be capable of producing lung damage. The lowest inflation pressure compatible with adequate chest wall expansion should therefore be used. Sometimes, however, pressures in excess of $30 \, cmH_2O$ will be necessary to inflate the surfactant-deficient lungs.

Pharyngeal suction

- Rarely necessary unless amniotic fluid stained with meconium or blood and the baby asphyxiated
- Can delay onset of spontaneous respiration for a long time if suction is aggressive
- Not recommended by direct mouth suction or oral mucus extractors because of congenital infection

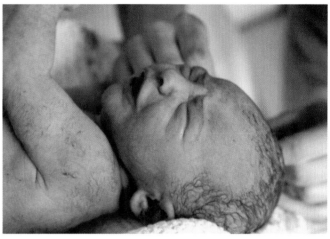

The goal of all deliveries—a healthy new born baby. With permission from Steve Percival/Science Photo Library

Further reading

- International guidelines 2000 for cardiopulmonary resuscitation and emergency cardiac care—a consensus on science. Part 11 neonatal resuscitation. *Resuscitation* 2000;46:401-6.
- Niermeyer S, Kattwinkel J, Van Reempts P, Nadkarni V, Philips B, Zideman D, et al. International guidelines for neonatal resuscitation: an excerpt from the guidelines 2000 for cardiopulmonary resuscitation and emergency cardiac care: Contributors and reviewers for the neonatal resuscitation guidelines. *Pediatrics* 2000;106:E29.
- Ellemunter H, Simma B, Trawoger R, Maurer H. Intraosseous lines in preterm and full term neonates. *Arch Dis Child* 1999;80:F74-F75.
- Field DJ, Milner AD, Hopkin IE. Efficacy of manual resuscitation at birth. *Arch Dis Child* 1986;61:300-2.
- Saugstad OD, Roorwelt T, Aalen O. Resuscitation of asphyxiated newborn infants with room air or oxygen: an international controlled trial: the Resair 2 Study. *Pediatrics* 1998:102:e1.
- Saugstad OD. Mechanisms of tissue injury by oxygen radicals: implications for neonatal disease. *Acta Pediatr* 1996;85:1-4.
- Vyas H, Field DJ, Milner AD, Hopkin IE. Physiological responses to prolonged and slow rise inflation. *J Pediatr* 1981;99:635-9.

10   Resuscitation of infants and children

David A Zideman, Kenneth Spearpoint

The aetiology of cardiac arrest in infants and children is different from that in adults. Infants and children rarely have primary cardiac events. In infants the commonest cause of death is sudden infant death syndrome, and in children aged between 1 and 14 years trauma is the major cause of death. In these age groups a primary problem is found with the airway. The resulting difficulties in breathing and the associated hypoxia rapidly cause severe bradycardia or asystole. The poor long-term outcome from many cardiac arrests in childhood is related to the severity of cellular anoxia that has to occur before the child's previously healthy heart succumbs. Organs sensitive to anoxia, such as the brain and kidney, may be severely damaged before the heart stops. In such cases cardiopulmonary resuscitation (CPR) may restore cardiac output but the child will still die from multisystem failure in the ensuing days, or the child may survive with serious neurological or systemic organ damage. Therefore, the early recognition of the potential for cardiac arrest, the prevention and limitation of serious injury, and earlier recognition of severe illness is clearly a more effective approach in children.

Paediatric basic life support

Early diagnosis and aggressive treatment of respiratory or cardiac insufficiency, aimed at avoiding cardiac arrest, are the keys to improving survival without neurological deficit in seriously ill children. Establishment of a clear airway and oxygenation are the most important actions in paediatric resuscitation. These actions are prerequisites for other forms of treatment.

Resuscitation should begin immediately without waiting for the arrival of equipment. This is essential in infants and children because clearing the airway may be all that is required. Assessment and treatment should proceed simultaneously to avoid losing vital time. As in any resuscitation event, the Airway-Breathing-Circulation sequence is the most appropriate.

If aspiration of a foreign body is strongly suspected, because of sudden onset of severe obstruction of the upper airway, the steps outlined in the section on choking should be taken immediately.

Assess responsiveness
Determine responsiveness by carefully stimulating the child. If the child is unresponsive, shout for help. Move the child only if he or she is in a dangerous location.

Airway
Open the airway by tilting the head and lifting the lower jaw. Care must be taken not to overextend the neck (as this may cause the soft trachea to kink and obstruct) and not to press on the soft tissues in the floor of the mouth. Pressure in this area will force the tongue into the airway and cause obstruction. The small infant is an obligatory nose breather so the patency of the nasal passages must be checked and maintained. Alternatively, the jaw thrust manoeuvre can be used when a

---

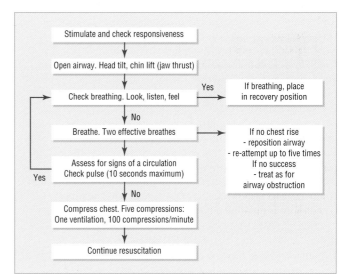

Algorithm for paediatric basic life support

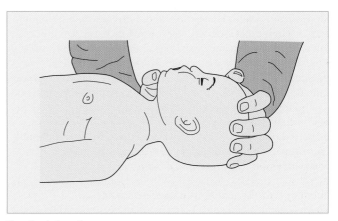

Opening infant airway

43

history of trauma or damage to the cervical spine is suspected. Maintaining the paediatric airway is a matter of trying various positions until the most satisfactory one is found. Rescuers must be flexible and willing to adapt their techniques.

Breathing

Assess breathing for 10 seconds while keeping the airway open by:

- Looking for chest and abdominal movement
- Listening at the mouth and nose for breath sounds
- Feeling for expired air movement with your cheek.

If the child's chest and abdomen are moving but no air can be heard or felt, the airway is obstructed. Readjust the airway and consider obstruction by a foreign body. If the child is not breathing, expired air resuscitation must be started immediately. With the airway held open, the rescuer covers the child's mouth (or mouth and nose for an infant) with their mouth and breathes out gently into the child until the chest is seen to rise. Minimise gastric distension by optimising the alignment of the airway and giving slow and steady inflations. Give two effective breaths, each lasting about 1-1.5 seconds, and note any signs of a response (the child may cough or "gag"). Up to five attempts may be made to achieve two effective breaths when the chest is seen to rise and fall.

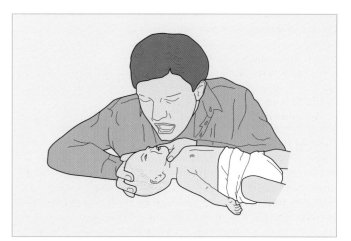

Mouth-to-mouth and nose ventilation

Circulation

Recent evidence has questioned the reliability of using a pulse check to determine whether effective circulation is present. Therefore, the rescuer should observe the child for 10 seconds for "signs of a circulation." This includes any movement, coughing, or breathing (more than an odd occasional gasp). In addition, healthcare providers are expected to check for the presence, rate, and volume of the pulse. The brachial pulse is easiest to feel in infants, whereas for children use the carotid pulse. The femoral pulse is an alternative for either. If none of the signs of a circulation have been detected, then start chest compressions without further delay and combine with ventilation. Immediate chest compressions, combined with ventilation, will also be indicated when a healthcare provider detects a pulse rate lower than 60 beats/min.

In infants and children the heart lies under the lower third of the sternum. In infants, compress the lower third of the sternum with two fingers of one hand; the upper finger should be one finger's breadth below an imaginary line joining the nipples. When more than one healthcare provider is present, the two-thumbed (chest encirclement) method of chest compression can be used for infants. The thumbs are aligned one finger's breadth below an imaginary line joining the nipples, the fingers encircle the chest, and the hands and fingers support the infant's rib cage and back. In children, the heel of one hand is positioned over a compression point two fingers' breadth above the xiphoid process. In both infants and children the sternum is compressed to about one third of the resting chest diameter; the rate is 100 compressions/min. The ratio of compressions to ventilations should be 5:1, irrespective of the number of rescuers. The compression phase should occupy half of the cycle and should be smooth, not jerky.

In larger, older children (over the age of eight years) the adult two-handed method of chest compression is normally used (see Chapter 1). The compression rate is 100/min and the compression to ventilation ratio is 15:2, but the compression depth changes to 4-5 cm.

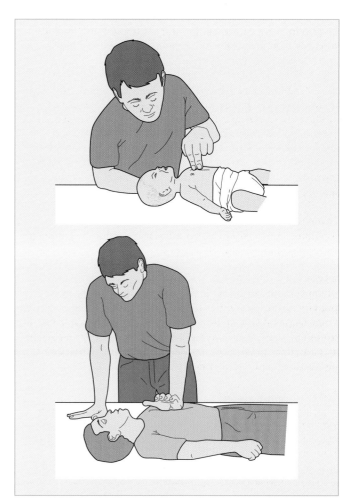

Chest compression in infants and children

Activation of the emergency medical services

When basic life support is being provided by a lone rescuer the emergency medical services must be activated after one minute because the provision of advanced life support procedures is vital to the child's survival. The single rescuer may be able to carry an infant or small child to the telephone, but older children will have to be left. Basic life support must be restarted as soon as possible after telephoning and continued without further interruption until advanced life support arrives. In circumstances in which additional help is available or the child has known heart disease, then the emergency medical services should be activated without delay.

Activate emergency services after one minute.

Choking

If airway obstruction caused by aspiration of a foreign body is witnessed or strongly suspected, special measures to clear the airway must be undertaken. Encourage the child, who is conscious and is breathing spontaneously, to cough and clear the obstruction themselves. Intervention is only necessary if these attempts are clearly ineffective and respiration is inadequate. Never perform blind finger sweeps of the pharynx because these can impact a foreign body in the larynx. Use measures intended to create a sharp increase in pressure within the chest cavity, such as an artificial cough.

Back blows

Hold the infant or child in a prone position and deliver up to five blows to the middle of the back between the shoulder blades. The head must be lower than the chest during this manoeuvre. This can be achieved by holding a small infant along the forearm or, for older children, across the thighs.

Chest thrusts

Place the child in a supine position. Give up to five thrusts to the sternum. The technique of chest thrusts is similar to that for chest compressions. The chest thrusts should be sharper and more vigorous than compressions and carried out at a slower rate of 20/min.

Check mouth

Remove any visible foreign bodies.

Open airway

Reposition the head by the head tilt and chin lift or jaw thrust manoeuvre and reassess air entry.

Breathe

Attempt rescue breathing if there are no signs of effective spontaneous respiration or if the airway remains obstructed. It may be possible to ventilate the child by positive pressure expired air ventilation when the airway is partially obstructed, but care must be taken to ensure that the child exhales most of this artificial ventilation after each breath.

Repeat

If the above procedure is unsuccessful in infants it should be repeated until the airway is cleared and effective respiration established. In children, abdominal thrusts are substituted for chest thrusts after the second round of back blows. Subsequently, back blows are combined with chest thrusts or abdominal thrusts in alternate cycles until the airway is cleared.

Paediatric advanced life support

The use of equipment in paediatric resuscitation is fraught with difficulties. Not only must a wide range be available to correspond with different sized infants and children but the rescuer must also choose and use each piece accurately.

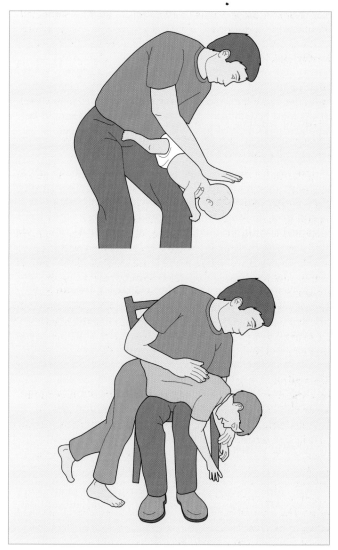

Back blows for choking infants and children are delivered between the shoulder blades with the subject prone

---

Abdominal thrusts

- In children over one year deliver up to five abdominal thrusts after the second five back blows. Use the upright position (Heimlich manoeuvre) if the child is conscious
- Unconscious children must be laid supine and the heel of one hand placed in the middle of the upper abdomen. Up to five sharp thrusts should be directed upwards toward the diaphragm
- Abdominal thrusts are not recommended in infants because they may cause damage to the abdominal viscera

ABC of Resuscitation

Effective basic life support is a prerequisite for successful advanced life support.

Airway and ventilation management

Airway and ventilation management is particularly important in infants and children during resuscitation because airway and respiratory problems are often the cause of the collapse. The airway must be established and the infant or child should be ventilated with high concentrations of inspired oxygen.

Airway adjuncts

Use an oropharyngeal (Guedel) airway if the child's airway cannot be maintained adequately by positioning alone during bag-valve-mask ventilation. A correctly sized airway should extend from the centre of the mouth to the angle of the jaw when laid against the child's face. A laryngeal mask can be used for those experienced in the technique.

Tracheal intubation is the definitive method of securing the airway. The technique facilitates ventilation and oxygenation and prevents pulmonary aspiration of gastric contents, but it does require training and practice. A child's larynx is narrower and shorter than that of any adult and the epiglottis is relatively longer and more U-shaped. The larynx is also in a higher, more anterior, and more acutely angled position than in the adult. A straight-bladed laryngoscope and plain plastic uncuffed tracheal tubes are therefore used in infants and young children. In children aged over one year the appropriate size of tracheal tube can be assessed by the following formula:

Internal diameter (mm) = (age in years/4) + 4

Infants in the first few weeks of life usually require a tube of size 3-3.5 mm, increasing to a size 4 when aged six to nine months.

Basic life support must not be interrupted for more than 30 seconds during intubation attempts. After this interval the child must be reoxygenated before a further attempt is made. If intubation cannot be achieved rapidly and effectively at this stage it should be delayed until later in the advanced life support protocol. Basic life support must continue.

Oxygenation and ventilation adjuncts

A flowmeter capable of delivering 15 l/min should be attached to the oxygen supply from either a central wall pipeline or an independent oxygen cylinder. Facemasks for mouth-to-mask or bag-valve-mask ventilation should be made of soft clear plastic, have a low dead space, and conform to the child's face to form a good seal. The circular design of facemask is recommended, especially when used by the inexperienced resuscitator. The facemask should be attached to a self-inflating bag-valve-mask of either 500 ml or 1600 ml capacity. The smaller bag size has a pressure-limiting valve attached to limit the maximum airway pressure to 30-35 cm H_2O and thus prevent pulmonary damage. Occasionally, this pressure-limiting valve may need to be overridden if the child has poorly compliant lungs. An oxygen reservoir system must be attached to the bag-valve-mask system, thereby enabling high inspired oxygen concentrations of over 80% to be delivered. The Ayre's T-piece with the open-ended bag (Jackson Reece modification) is not recommended because it requires specialist training to be able to operate it safely and effectively.

Management protocols for advanced life support

Having established an airway and effective ventilation with high inspired oxygen, the next stage of the management depends on the cardiac rhythm. The infant or child must therefore be attached to a cardiac monitor or its electrocardiogram (ECG) monitored through the paddles of a defibrillator.

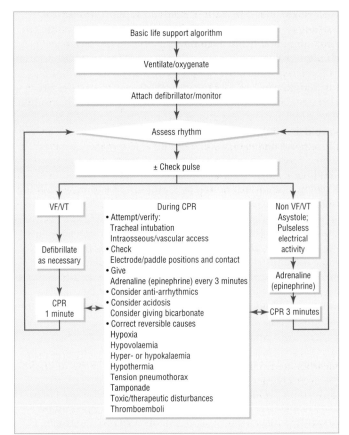

Algorithm for paediatric advanced life support

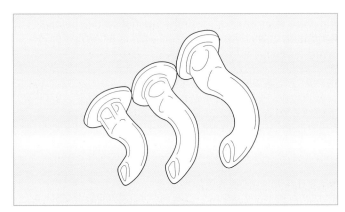

Guedel oropharyngeal airways

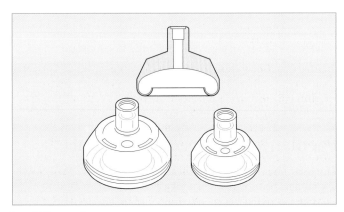

Laerdal face masks

Non-ventricular fibrillation/non-ventricular tachycardia

Asystole is the commonest cardiac arrest rhythm in infancy and childhood. It is the final common pathway of respiratory or circulatory failure and is usually preceded by an agonal bradycardia.

The diagnosis of asystole is made on electrocardiographic evidence in a pulseless patient. Care must be taken to ensure that the electrocardiograph leads are correctly positioned and attached and that the monitor gain is turned up. Effective basic life support and ventilation with high-flow oxygen through a patent airway are essential. Having established a secure airway and intravenous or intraosseous access, 10 mcg/kg (0.1 ml/kg of 1:10 000) of adrenaline (epinephrine) is administered followed by three minutes of basic life support. If asystole persists then a further dose of 0.1 ml/kg of 1:10 000 adrenaline (epinephrine) should be administered during the subsequent three minute period of CPR. If asystole persists, further three-minute sequences of CPR with adrenaline (epinephrine) at doses of 10-100 mcg/kg (0.1 ml/kg of 1:1000) may be given while considering other drugs and interventions.

Alkalising agents are of unproven benefit and should be used only after clinical diagnosis of profound acidosis in patients with respiratory or circulatory arrest if the first dose of adrenaline (epinephrine) has been ineffective. The dose of bicarbonate is 1 mmol/kg and is given as a single bolus by slow intravenous injection, ideally before the second dose of adrenaline (epinephrine). If an alkalising agent is used then the cannula must be thoroughly flushed with normal saline before any subsequent dosing with adrenaline (epinephrine) because this drug will be chemically inactivated by the alkalising agent. Subsequent treatment with alkalising agents should be guided by the blood pH.

A bolus of normal saline should follow the intravenous or intraosseous injection of any drug used in resuscitation, especially if the injection site is peripheral. The amount should be 5-20 ml, depending on the size of the child. When cardiac arrest has resulted from circulatory failure a larger bolus of fluid should be given if no response or only a poor response to the initial dose of adrenaline (epinephrine) is seen. Examples of such cases are children with hypovolaemia from blood loss, gastroenteritis, or sepsis when a profound distributive hypovolaemic shock may occur. These children require 20 ml/kg of a crystalloid (normal saline or Ringer's lactate) or a colloid (5% human albumin or an artificial colloid).

Pulseless electrical activity

Formerly known as electromechanical dissociation, pulseless electrical activity (PEA) is described as a normal (or near normal) ECG in the absence of a detectable pulse. If not treated, this rhythm will soon degenerate through agonal bradycardia to asystole. It is managed in the same way as asystole, with oxygenation and ventilation accompanying basic life support and adrenaline (epinephrine) to support coronary and cerebral perfusion.

Ventricular fibrillation and pulseless ventricular tachycardia

Ventricular fibrillation is relatively rare in children, but it is occasionally seen in cardiothoracic intensive care units or in patients being investigated for congenital heart disease. In contrast to the treatment of asystole, defibrillation takes precedence. Defibrillation is administered in a series of three energy shocks followed by one minute of basic life support. The defibrillation energy is 2 J/kg for the first shock, 2 J/kg for the second rising to 4 J/kg for the third and all subsequent defibrillation attempts. For defibrillators with

Two arrest rhythms

- Non-VF/VT: asystole or pulseless electrical activity
- Ventricular fibrillation or pulseless ventricular tachycardia

Asystole

- Common arrest rhythm in children
- ECG evidence in a pulseless patient

Asystole in an infant or child

PEA

- Absence of cardiac output with normal or near normal ECG
- ECG evidence in pulseless patient

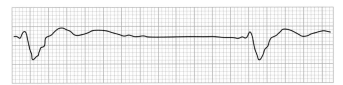

Broad and slow rhythm is associated with pulseless electrical activity

Ventricular fibrillation and pulseless ventricular tachycardia

- Characteristic ECG in pulseless patient
- Relatively rare in children
- Treatment is immediate defibrillation

stepped current levels the nearest higher step to the calculated energy level required should be selected.

Ventilation and chest compressions should be continued at all times except when shocks are being delivered or the ECG is being studied for evidence of change. Paediatric paddles should be used in children below 10 kg, but in bigger children the larger adult electrode will minimise transthoracic impedance and should be used when the child's thorax is broad enough to permit electrode-to-chest contact over the entire paddle surface. One paddle should be placed over the apex of the heart and one beneath the right clavicle. Alternatively, a front-to-back position can be used.

Consider giving adrenaline (epinephrine) every three minutes during resuscitation. In ventricular fibrillation adrenaline (epinephrine) should be administered as 10 mcg/kg initially followed by 10-100 mcg/kg for all subsequent administrations.

Other considerations

As mentioned previously, it is rare for infants and children to have a primary cardiac arrest. Therefore, it is important to seek out and treat the initial cause of the cardiorespiratory collapse. This cause should be sought while basic and advanced life support continues. The most common causes can be summarised as the 4Hs and 4Ts.

When detected, the underlying cause must be treated rapidly and appropriately.

4Hs and 4Ts

- Hypoxia
- Hypovolaemia
- Hyper- or hypokalaemia
- Hypothermia
- Tension pneumothorax
- Tamponade
- Toxic or therapeutic disturbances
- Thromboembolism

Drug doses and equipment sizes

An important consideration when managing cardiac arrest in children is the correct estimation of drug doses, fluid volumes, and equipment sizes. There are two systems in current use. The first entails a calculation based on the length of the child and a specifically designed tape measure (the Broselow tape. The other uses a length-weight-age nomogram chart (the Oakley chart). It is important to become familiar with and to use one of these systems.

Audit of results

The future development of paediatric guidelines will be determined by an examination of published scientific evidence. The Utstein Template has aided the uniform collection of data from paediatric resuscitation attempts.

Drugs and fluid administration

If venous access has not been established before the cardiorespiratory collapse, peripheral venous access should be attempted. This is notoriously difficult in small ill children. Central venous access is also difficult except in the hands of experts, is hazardous in children, and is unlikely to provide a more rapid route for drugs. If venous access is not gained within 90 seconds, the intraosseous route should be attempted.

Endotracheal tube

Oral length (cm)	Internal diameter (mm)
18-21	7.5-8.0 (cuffed)
18	7.0 (uncuffed)
17	6.5
16	6.0
15	5.5
14	5.0
13	4.5
12	4.0
	3.5
10	3.0-3.5

	Weight	5	10	20	30	40	50 kg
Adrenaline/epinephrine (ml of 1 in 10 000) intravenous or intraosseous		0.5	1	2	3	4	5
Adrenaline/epinephrine (ml of 1 in 1000) endotracheal		0.5	1	2	3	4	5
*Atropine (ml of 100μg/ml) intravenous or intraosseous		1	2	4	6	8	10
Atropine (ml of 600μg/ml)		-	0.3	0.7	1	1.3	1.7
*Amiodarone (ml of 30μg/ml prefilled) (bolus in cardiac arrest, slowly over 3 minutes if not) intravenous or intraosseous		0.8	1.5	3.5	5	6.5	8.5ml
			dilute appropriately in 5% glucose				
*Amiodarone (ml of 50μg/ml concentrated solution)		0.5	1	2	3	4	5ml
			dilute appropriately in 5% glucose				
*Bicarbonate (mmol) intravenous or intraosseous		5	10	20	30	40	50 mmol
*Calcium chloride (ml of 10%) intravenous or intraosseous		0.5	1	2	3	4	5
*Lidocaine/lignocaine (ml of 1%) intravenous or intraosseous		0.5	1	2	3	4	5
Initial DC defibrillation (J) for ventricular fibrillation or pulseless ventricular tachycardia		10	20	40	60	80	100J
Initial DC cardioversion (J) for supraventricular tachycardia with shock (synchronous) or ventricular tachycardia with shock (non-synchronous)		5	5	10	15	20	25J
**Initial fluid bolus in shock (ml) intravenous or intraosseous (crystalloid or colloid)		100	200	400	600	800	1000
Glucose (ml of 10%) intravenous or intraosseous		25	50	100	150	200	250
Lorazepam (ml of 5mg diluted to 5ml in 0.9% saline) intravenous or intraosseous		0.5	1	2	3	4	5
Lorazepam (ml of 5mg/ml neat)		-	-	0.4	0.6	0.8	1
Diazepam (mg rectal tube solution) (if lorazepam or intravenous access not available) rectal		2.5	5	10	10	10	10mg
Naloxone neonatal (ml of 20μg/ml) intravenous or intraosseous		2.5	5	-	-	-	-
Naloxone adult (ml of 400μg/ml)		-	0.25	0.5	0.75	1	1.25
*Salbutamol (mg nebuliser solution) by nebuliser (dilute to 2.5-5 ml in physiological saline)		-	2.5	5	5	5	5mg

* Caution! Non-standard drug concentrations may be available:
Use atropine 100 μg/ml or prepare by diluting 1 mg to 10 ml or 600 μg to 6 ml in 0.9% saline
Bicarbonate is available in various concentrations (8.4% has 1 mmol/ml; 4.2% has 0.5 mmol/ml; 1.26% has 0.15 mmol/ml). In infants, avoid 8.4% or dilute to at least 4.2%.
Note that 1 ml of calcium chloride 10% is equivalent to 3 ml of calcium gluconate 10%
Use lidocaine/lignocaine (*without* adrenaline/epinephrine) 1% or give half the volume of 2% (or dilute appropriately)
In the initial nebulised dose of salbutamol, ipratropium may be added to the nebuliser in doses of 250 μg for a 10 kg child and 500 μg for an older child. Salbutamol may also be given by slow intravenous injection (5 μg/kg over 5 minutes), but beware of the different concentrations available (eg 50 and 500 μg/ml)
** In uncontrolled haemorrhage, give fluid in careful, repeated increments (eg 5 ml/kg rather than 20 ml/kg at once) to maintain a palpable pulse and minimum acceptable blood pressure until bleeding is controlled

The Oakley chart

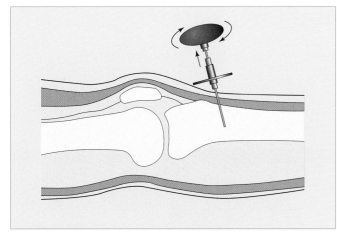

Intraosseous infusion needle placed in the upper tibia

Further reading

● APLS Working Group. *Advanced paediatric life support. The practical approach.* 3rd ed. London: BMJ Publishing Group, 2001.
● European Resuscitation Council. Guidelines 2000 for cardiopulmonary resuscitation and cardiovascular care—an international consensus on science. *Resuscitation* 2000;46:301-400.
● Nadkarni V, Hazinski MF, Zideman DA, Kattwinkel K, Quan L, Bingham R, et al. Paediatric life support: an advisory statement by the Paediatric Life Support Working Group of the International Liaison Committee on Resuscitation. *Resuscitation* 1997;34:115-27.
● Luten R, Wears R, Broselow J, Zaritsky A, Barnett T, Lee T. Length based endotracheal tube and emergency equipment selection in paediatrics. *Ann Emerg Med* 1992;2:900-4.
● Oakley P. Inaccuracy and delay in decision making in paediatric resuscitation and a proposed reference chart to reduce error. *BMJ* 1988;297:817-9.
● Oakley P, Phillips B, Molyneux E, Mackway-Jones K. Paediatric resuscitation. *BMJ* 1994;306:1613.
● Zaritsky A, Nadkarni V, Hanzinski MF, Foltin G, Quan L, Wright J, et al. Recommended guidelines for uniform reporting of paediatric advanced life support: the paediatric utstein style. *Resuscitation* 1995;30:95-116.

Intraosseous access is a safe, simple, and rapid means of circulatory access for infants and children. Resuscitation drugs, fluid, and blood can be safely given via this route and rapidly reach the heart. Complications are uncommon and usually result from prolonged use of the site or poor technique. Marrow aspirate can be drawn and used to estimate concentrations of haemoglobin, sodium, potassium, chloride, glucose, venous pH, and blood groups.

If circulatory access proves impossible to achieve within two to three minutes, some drugs, including adrenaline (epinephrine) and atropine, can be given down the tracheal tube. Data from studies on animals and humans suggest that the endotracheal dose of adrenaline (epinephrine) should be 10 times the standard dose, but doubts have been cast on the reliability of this route and intravenous or intraosseous drug administration is preferable.

The algorithms for paediatric basic life support and paediatric advanced life support are adapted from *Resuscitation Guidelines 2000*, London: Resuscitation Council (UK), 2000. The diagrams of Guedel oropharyngeal airways and Laerdal masks are adapted from *Newborn Life Support Manual*, London: Resuscitation Council (UK). The diagram of and intraosseous infusion needle is courtesy of Cook Critical Care (UK).

11   Resuscitation in the ambulance service

Andrew K Marsden

Sudden death outside hospital is common. In England alone, more than 50 000 medically unattended deaths occur each year. The survival of countless patients with acute myocardial infarction, primary cardiac arrhythmia, trauma, or vascular catastrophe is threatened by the lack of immediate care outside hospital. The case for providing prompt and effective resuscitation at the scene of an emergency is overwhelming, but only comparatively recently has this subject begun to receive the attention it deserves.

Development

The origin of the modern ambulance can be traced to Baron von Larrey, a young French army surgeon who, in 1792, devised a light vehicle to take military surgeons and their equipment to the front battle lines of the Napoleonic wars. Larrey's walking carts or horse-drawn ambulances volantes ("flying ambulances") were the forerunners of the sophisticated mobile intensive care units of today.

The delivery of emergency care to patients before admission to hospital started in Europe in the 1960s. Professor Frank Pantridge pioneered a mobile coronary care unit in Belfast in 1966, and he is generally credited with introducing the concept of "bringing hospital treatment to the community." He showed that resuscitation vehicles crewed by medical or nursing staff could effectively treat patients with sudden illness or trauma.

The use of emergency vehicles carrying only paramedic staff, who were either in telephone contact with a hospital or acting entirely without supervision, was explored in the early 1970s, most extensively in the United States. The Medic 1 scheme started in Seattle in 1970 by Dr Leonard Cobb used the fire tenders of a highly coordinated fire service that could reach an emergency in any part of the city within four minutes. All firefighters were trained in basic life support and defibrillation and were supported by well-equipped Medic 1 ambulances crewed by paramedics with at least 12 months full-time training in emergency care.

In the United Kingdom the development of civilian paramedic schemes was slow. The Brighton experiment in ambulance training began in 1971 and schemes in other centres followed independently over the next few years. It was only due to individual enthusiasm (by pioneers like Baskett, Chamberlain, and Ward) and private donations for equipment that any progress was made. A pilot course of extended training in ambulance was launched after the Miller Report (1966-1967) and recognition by the Department of Health of the value of pre-hospital care. Three years later, after industrial action by the ambulance service, the then Minister of Health, Kenneth Clarke, pronounced that paramedics with extended training should be included in every emergency ambulance call, and he made funding available to provide each front-line ambulance with a defibrillator.

In Scotland an extensive fundraising campaign enabled advisory defibrillators to be placed in each of the 500 emergency vehicles by the middle of 1990 and a

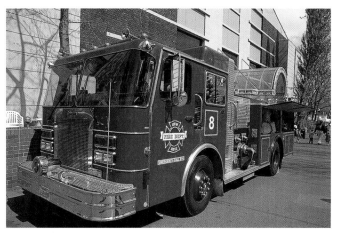
Seattle fire truck

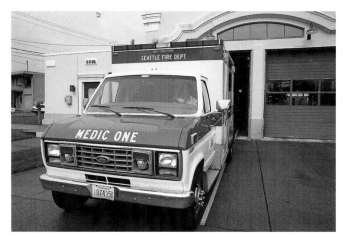
Seattle ambulance

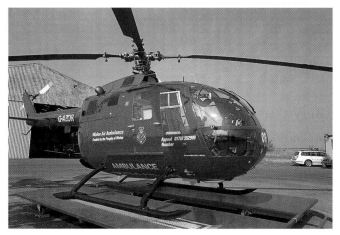
A helicopter is used to speed the response

sophisticated programme ("Heartstart Scotland") was initiated to review the outcome of every ambulance resuscitation attempt.

Chain of survival

The ambulance service is able to make useful contributions to each of the links in the chain of survival that is described in Chapter 1.

Early awareness and early access

The United Kingdom has had a dedicated emergency call number (999) to access the emergency services since 1937. In Europe, a standard emergency call number (112) is available and a number of countries, including the United Kingdom, respond to this as well as to their usual national emergency number.

All ambulance services in the United Kingdom now employ a system of prioritised despatch, either Advanced Medical Priority Despatch or Criteria Based Despatch, in which the call-taker follows a rigorously applied algorithm to ensure that the urgency of the problem is identified according to defined criteria and that the appropriate level of response is assigned.

Three categories of call are usually recognised:

- Category A—Life threatening (including cardiopulmonary arrest). The aim is to get to most of these calls within eight minutes
- Category B—Emergency but not immediately life threatening
- Category C—Non-urgent. An appropriate response is provided; in some cases the transfer of the call is transferred to other agencies, such as NHS Direct.

Having assigned a category to the call (often with the help of a computer algorithm), the call-taker will pass it to a dispatcher who, using appropriate technology such as automated vehicle location systems, will ask the nearest ambulance or most appropriate resource to respond. In the case of cardiorespiratory arrest this may also include a community first responder who can be rapidly mobilised with an automated defibrillator.

The ambulance control room staff will also provide emergency advice to the telephone caller, including instructions on how to perform cardiopulmonary resuscitation if appropriate.

The speed of response is critical because survival after cardiorespiratory arrest falls exponentially with time. The Heartstart Scotland scheme has shown that those patients who develop ventricular fibrillation after the arrival of the ambulance crew have a greater than 50% chance of long-term survival.

The ambulance controller should ensure that patients with suspected myocardial infarction are also attended promptly by their general practitioner. Such a "dual response" provides the patient with effective analgesia, electrocardiographic monitoring, defibrillation, and advanced life support as soon as possible. It also allows pre-hospital thrombolysis.

Early cardiopulmonary resuscitation

The benefits of early cardiopulmonary resuscitation have been well established, with survival from all forms of cardiac arrest at least doubled when bystander cardiopulmonary resuscitation is undertaken. All emergency service staff should be trained in effective basic life support and their skills should be regularly refreshed and updated. In most parts of the United Kingdom ambulance staff also train the general public in emergency life support techniques.

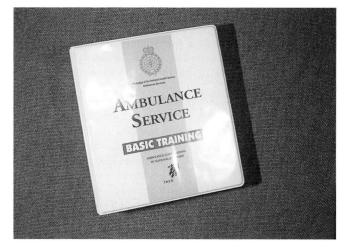
NHS Training Manual

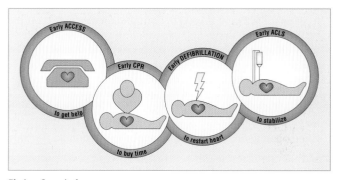
Chain of survival

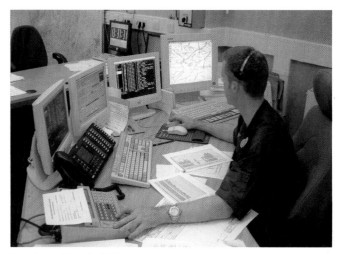
Ambulance dispatch desk

Early defibrillation

Every front-line ambulance in the United Kingdom now carries a defibrillator, most often an advisory or automated external defibrillator (AED) that can be used by all grades of ambulance staff.

The results of early defibrillation with AEDs operated by ambulance staff are encouraging. In Scotland alone, where currently over 35 000 resuscitation attempts are logged on the database, 16 500 patients have been defibrillated since 1988, with almost 1800 long-term survivors—that is, 150 survivors per year—an overall one year survival rate from out-of-hospital ventricular fibrillation of about 10%.

The introduction of AEDs has revolutionised defibrillation outside hospital. The sensitivity and specificity of these defibrillators is comparable to manual defibrillators and the time taken to defibrillate is less. AEDs have high-quality data recording, retrieval, and analysis systems and, most importantly, potential users become competent in their use after considerably less training. The development of AEDs has extended the availability of defibrillation to any first responder, not only ambulance staff (see Chapter 3). It is nevertheless important that such first responder schemes, which often include the other emergency services or the first aid societies, are integrated into a system with overall medical control usually coordinated by the ambulance service.

Early advanced life support

The standardised course used to train paramedics builds on the substantial basic training and experience given to ambulance technicians. It emphasises the extended skills of venous cannulation, recording and interpreting electrocardiograms (ECGs), intubation, infusion, defibrillation, and the use of selected drugs. In 1992 the Medicines Act was amended to permit ambulance paramedics to administer approved drugs from a range of prescription only medicines.

The paramedic training course covers, in a modular form, the theoretical and practical knowledge needed for the extended care of emergency conditions in a minimum instruction time of 400 hours. Four weeks of the course is provided in hospital under the supervision of clinical tutors in cardiology, accident and emergency medicine, anaesthesia, and intensive care. Training in emergency paediatrics and obstetric care (including neonatal resuscitation) is also provided. All grades of ambulance staff are subject to review and audit as part of the clinical governance arrangements operated by Ambulance Trusts. Paramedics must refresh their skills annually and attend a residential intensive revision course at an approved centre every three years. Opportunities are also provided for further hospital placement if necessary.

The ability to provide early advanced life support techniques other than defibrillation—for example, advanced airway care and ventilation—probably contributes to the overall success of ambulance based resuscitation. The precise role of the ambulance service in delivering advanced life support remains controversial, but the overwhelming impression is that paramedics considerably enhance the professional image of the service and the quality of patient care provided.

Coordination and audit

Local enthusiasm remains a cornerstone for developing resuscitation within the ambulance service, but growing interest from the Department of Health and senior ambulance

Equipment for front-line ambulance
- Immediate response satchel—bag, valve, mask (adult and child), hand-held suction, airways, laryngoscopy roll, endotracheal tubes, dressing pads, scissors
- Portable oxygen therapy set
- Portable ventilator
- Defibrillator and monitor and accessories, pulse oximeter
- Sphygmomanometer and stethoscope
- Entonox
- Trolley cots, stretchers, poles, pillows, blankets
- Rigid collars
- Vacuum splints
- Spine immobiliser, long spine board
- Fracture splints
- Drug packs, intravenous fluids, and cannulas
- Waste bins, sharps box
- Maternity pack
- Infectious diseases pack
- Hand lamp
- Rescue tools

Drugs sanctioned for use by trained ambulance staff
- Oxygen
- Entonox
- Aspirin
- Nitroglycerine
- Adrenaline (epinephrine) 1:10 000
- Lignocaine
- Atropine
- Diazepam
- Salbutamol
- Glucagon
- Naxloxone
- Nalbuphine
- Syntometrine
- Sodium bicarbonate
- Glucose infusion
- Saline infusion
- Ringer's lactate infusion
- Polygeline infusion
- Metoclopramide
- Frusemide
- Morphine sulphate
- Benzyl penicillin

Outline syllabus for paramedic training
Theoretical knowledge
Basic anatomy and physiology
- Respiratory system (especially mouth and larynx)
- Heart and circulation
- Central and autonomic nervous system
Presentation of common disorders
- Respiratory obstruction, distress, or failure
- Presentations of ischaemic heart disease
- Differential diagnosis of chest pain
- Complications and management of acute myocardial infarction
- Acute abdominal emergencies
- Open and closed injury of chest and abdomen
- Limb fractures
- Head injury
- Fitting
- Burns
- Maxillofacial injuries
- Obstetric care
- Paediatric emergencies
Practical skills
Observing and assessing patient
- Assessing the scene of the emergency
- Taking a brief medical history
- Observing general appearance, pulse, blood pressure (with sphygmomanometer), level of consciousness (with Glasgow scale)
- Undertaking systemic external examination for injury
- Recording and interpreting the ECG and rhythm monitor
Interventions
- Basic life support
- Defibrillation
- Intubation
- Vascular access
- Drug administration

authorities is now leading to greater central encouragement and coordination.

The Joint Royal Colleges' Ambulance Liaison Committee includes representatives from the Royal Colleges of Physicians, Surgeons, Anaesthetists, General Practitioners, Paediatricians, Nurses, and Midwives who meet regularly with representatives from the ambulance service and other professional groups. This body, and its equivalent in Scotland, the Professional Advisory Group, provide a strong voice for pre-hospital care based on a sound medical and professional footing.

Audit of resuscitation practice and outcomes using the Utstein template is an important component of ambulance resuscitation practice. To allow interservice comparisons, most services audit their performance against outcome criteria, such as the return of spontaneous circulation and survival to leave hospital alive.

The ambulance services now have their own professional association, the Ambulance Services Association, which sets and regulates ambulance standards, including evidence based guidelines for ambulance care. Lobbying from this group, together with representations from other groups, has now resulted in the formal "State Registration" of ambulance paramedics as professionals supplementary to medicine.

Benefits

The number of successful resuscitations each year is a relatively easy benefit to quantify. Rates at well established centres vary between 20 and 100 successful resuscitations each year for populations of about 350 000. Success in this context means discharge from hospital of an active, mentally alert patient who would otherwise have stood no chance of survival without pre-hospital care. Techniques that provide comfort and prevent complications are less readily assessed but may also be important.

The observed benefits of an ambulance service able to provide resuscitation skills

- Successful cardiopulmonary resuscitation
- Increasing awareness of the need for a rapid response to emergencies
- Improved monitoring and support of the critically ill
- Improved standard of care for non-urgent patients

Further reading

- National Health Service Training Directorate. *Ambulance service paramedic training manual.* Bristol: National Health Service Training Directorate, 1991.
- Cobbe SM, Redmond MJ, Watson JM, Hollingworth J, Carrington DJ. "Heartstart Scotland"—initial experience of a national scheme for out of hospital defibrillation. *BMJ* 1991;302:1517-20.
- Cummins RO, Ornato JP, Thies WH, Pepe PE. Improving survival from sudden cardiac arrest: the "chain of survival" concept. *Circulation* 1991;83:1832-47.
- Lewis SJ, Holmberg S, Quinn E, Baker K, Grainger R, Vincent R, et al. Out of hospital resuscitation in East Sussex, 1981-1989. *Br Heart J* 1993;70:568-73.
- Mackintosh A, Crabb ME, Granger R, Williams JH, Chamberlain DA. The Brighton resuscitation ambulances: review of 40 consecutive survivors of out of hospital cardiac arrest. *BMJ* 1978;i:1115-8.
- Partridge JF, Adgey AA, Geddes JS, Webb SW. *The acute coronary attack.* Tunbridge Wells: Pitman Medical, 1975.
- Sedgwick ML, Watson J, Dalziel K, Carrington DJ, Cobbe SM. Efficacy of out of hospital defibrillation by ambulance technicians using automatic external defibrillators. The Heartstart Scotland project. *Resuscitation* 1991;24:73-87.

12 Resuscitation in hospital

T R Evans

Patients suffering a cardiac arrest in a British hospital have a one in three chance of initial successful resuscitation, a one in five chance of leaving hospital alive, and a one in seven chance of still being alive one year later. Younger patients and those nursed in a specialist area (such as a Cardiac Care Unit or accident and emergency department) at the time of cardiac arrest have a considerably better outlook, with about twice the chance of surviving one year. Any patient who suffers a cardiopulmonary arrest in hospital has the right to expect the maximum chance of survival because the staff should be appropriately trained and equipped in all aspects of resuscitation.

In specialist areas a fully equipped resuscitation trolley should always be on site with staff trained in advanced life support, preferably holding the Advanced Life Support Provider Certificate of the Resuscitation Council (UK). Every general ward should have its own defibrillator, usually an automated external defibrillator (AED), with the maximum number of staff, particularly nursing staff, trained to use it.

AEDs should also be available in other areas such as outpatients, physiotherapy, and radiology. The minimum requirement for any hospital must be to have one defibrillator and one resuscitation trolley on each clinical floor.

As a cardiac arrest can occur anywhere in the hospital, it is essential that as many as possible of the clerical, administrative, and other support staff should be trained in basic life support to render immediate assistance while awaiting the arrival of the cardiac arrest team.

Training of staff in cardiopulmonary resuscitation

All medical and nursing students should be required to show competence in basic life support, the use of basic airway adjuncts, and the use of an AED. Medical schools should run advanced life support courses for final year medical students, either over a three day period or on a modular basis. Students should have an advanced life support provider certificate approved by the Resuscitation Council (UK) before qualifying. If this cannot be achieved at the present time the intermediate life support course of the Resuscitation Council (UK), a one day course, should be considered.

All qualified medical and nursing personnel should possess the skills they are likely to have to practise in the event of a cardiorespiratory arrest, depending on their specialty and the role that they would have to take. The minimum requirement is basic life support plus training in the use of an AED. Staff should requalify at regular intervals, specified by the resuscitation committee of the hospital within the clinical governance protocols followed by their employing authority. Medical staff and nursing staff working in critical care areas or who form part of the resuscitation team should hold a current advanced life support provider certificate approved by the Resuscitation Council (UK). Staff dealing with children should possess a paediatric advanced life support certificate, and if

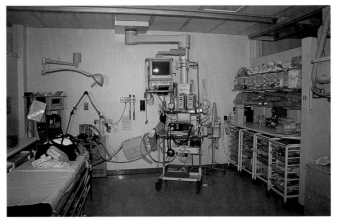

Adult resuscitation room in accident and emergency department

---

Hospital area types

Specialist
- Cardiac care
- Intensive care
- Emergency
- Operating theatres
- Specialist intervention areas—for example, catheterisation laboratories, endoscopy units

General
- Wards
- Departments—for example, physiotherapy, outpatients, radiology

Common parts
- The overall concourse areas

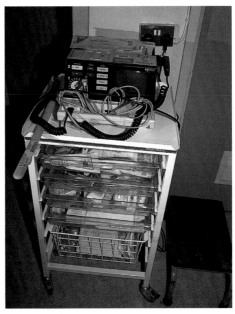

A defibrillation station should be prominent in areas of high risk

they deal with neonates they should hold a current provider certificate in neonatal resuscitation.

To maintain the standard of resuscitation in the hospital it is valuable to have a core of instructors to help run "in-house" courses and advise the resuscitation team. It is hoped that in the future the Royal Colleges will require evidence of advanced life support skills before permitting entry to higher medical diploma examinations. Some specialist training committees already require specialist registrars to possess an advanced life support certificate before specialist registration can be granted.

It is unacceptable to have to wait for the arrival of the cardiac arrest trolley on a general medical ward or in an area, such as outpatients, in which cardiac arrests may occur. Most survivors from cardiac arrest have developed a shockable rhythm, such as ventricular fibrillation or pulseless ventricular tachycardia, and may be successfully shocked before the arrival of the cardiac arrest team. The function of this team is then to provide advanced life support techniques, such as advanced airway management and drug therapy.

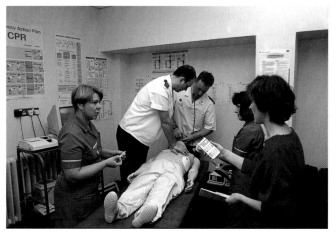

A cardiac arrest team training

The resuscitation committee

Every hospital should have a resuscitation committee as recommended in the Royal College of Physicians' report. Its composition will vary. The committee should ensure that hospital staff are appropriately and adequately trained, that there is sufficient resuscitation equipment in good working order throughout the hospital, and that adequate training facilities are available. The minutes of the committee's meetings should be sent to the medical director or appropriate medical executive or advisory committee of the hospital and should highlight any dangerous or deficient areas of practice, such as lack of equipment or properly trained staff. Postgraduate deans or tutors (or both) should be ex-officio members of the committee to facilitate liaison on training matters and to ensure that adequate time and money is set aside to allow junior doctors to receive training in resuscitation.

The resuscitation officer

The resuscitation officer should be an approved instructor in advanced life support, often also in paediatric advanced life support and sometimes in advanced trauma life support. The background of resuscitation officers is usually that of a nurse with several years' experience in a critical care unit, an operating department assistant, or a very experienced ambulance paramedic. The resuscitation officer is directly responsible to the chair of the resuscitation committee and receives full backing in carrying out the role as defined by that committee. It is essential that a dedicated resuscitation training room is available and that adequate secretarial help, a computer, telephone, fax machine, and office space are provided to enable the resuscitation officer to work efficiently. As well as conducting the in-hospital audit of resuscitation, he or she should be encouraged to undertake research studies to further their career development.

Doctors, nurses, and managers do not always recognise the crucial importance of having a resuscitation officer, especially when funding has been a major issue. Training should be mandatory for all staff undertaking general medical care. It is likely that many specialties will require formal training in cardiopulmonary resuscitation before a certificate of accreditation is granted in that specialty.

It is advisable that the recommendations of the Royal College of Physicians' report and the recommendations of the

The resuscitation committee

- Specialists in:
  Cardiology or general medicine
  Anaesthesia and critical care
  Emergency medicine
  Paediatrics
- Resuscitation officer
- Nursing staff representative
- Pharmacist
- Administrative and support staff representative—for example, porters
- Telephonists' representative

The resuscitation committee should receive a regular audit of resuscitation attempts, hold audit meetings, and take remedial action if it seems necessary. Resuscitation provision and performance should be regularly reviewed as part of the clinical governance process

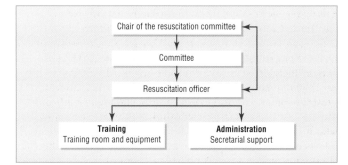

Resuscitation team structure

Resuscitation Council (UK) should be implemented in full in all hospitals. All hospitals should have a unique telephone number to be used in case of suspected cardiac arrest. It would be helpful if hospitals standardised this number (222 or 2222) so that staff moving from hospital to hospital do not have to learn a new number each time they move. This emergency number should be displayed prominently on every telephone. When the number is dialled an audible alarm should be sounded in the telephone room of the hospital, giving the call equal priority with a fire alarm call. Because the person instigating the call may not know exactly what location they are calling from, the telephone should indicate this—for example, "cardiac arrest, Jenner Hoskin ward, third floor." By pressing a single button in the telephone room all the cardiac arrest bleeps should be activated, indicating a cardiac arrest and its location.

The hospital resuscitation committee should determine the composition of the cardiac arrest team. In multistorey hospitals those carrying the cardiac bleep must have an override facility to commandeer the lifts.

The resuscitation officer must ensure that after any resuscitation attempt, the necessary documentation is accurately completed in "Utstein format." Nursing staff should check and restock the resuscitation trolley after every resuscitation attempt.

It is essential that the senior doctor and nurse at the cardiac arrest should debrief the team, whether resuscitation has been successful or not. Problems should be discussed frankly. If any member of staff is especially distressed then a confidential counselling facility should be made available through the occupational health or psychological medicine department.

Presence of relatives

It is now accepted by many resuscitation providers and institutions that the relatives of those who have suffered a cardiac arrest may wish to witness the resuscitation attempt. This applies particularly to the parents of children. Clear guidelines are available from the Resuscitation Council (UK) detailing how relatives should be supported during cardiopulmonary resuscitation procedures. Allowing relatives to witness resuscitation attempts seems, in many cases, to allow them to feel that everything possible has been done for their relative even if the attempt at resuscitation is unsuccessful, and may be a help in the grieving process.

Do not attempt resuscitation orders

For some patients, attempts at cardiopulmonary resuscitation are not appropriate because of the terminal nature of their illness or the futility of the attempt. Every hospital resuscitation committee should agree a "do not attempt resuscitation" (DNAR) policy with its ethics committee and medical advisory committee (see Chapter 21). In many cases it may be appropriate to discuss the suitability of attempting cardiopulmonary resuscitation with the patient or with his or her relatives in the light of the patient's diagnosis, the probability of success, and the likely quality of subsequent life.

When a competent person has expressed his or her views on resuscitation in a correctly executed and applicable advance directive or "living will," these wishes should be respected. DNAR orders and the reasons for them must be clearly documented in the medical notes and should be signed by the consultant in charge or, in his or her absence, by a doctor of at least specialist registrar grade. All such entries should be dated

---

The cardiac arrest team
- Specialist registrar or senior house officer in medicine
- Specialist registrar or senior house officer in anaesthesia
- Junior doctor
- Nursing staff
- Operating department assistant (optional)

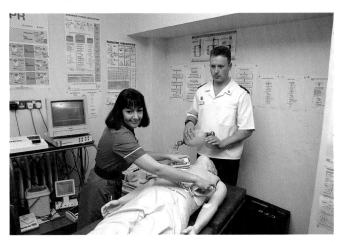

Practising in the resuscitation training room

The resuscitation training room

This room should be totally dedicated to resuscitation training and fully equipped with resuscitation manikins, arrhythmia simulators, intubation trainers, and other required training aids

---

DNAR orders
- Hospital's policy must be agreed with ethics and medical advisory committees
- Discuss with patients or relatives (or both) when appropriate
- Advance directive or "living will" views must be respected
- DNAR orders must be documented and signed by the doctor responsible
- All DNAR decisions must be discussed by staff involved
- All DNAR orders must be documented in nursing notes
- In the absence of a DNAR order cardiopulmonary resuscitation must be commenced
- Policy must be regularly reviewed

and the hospital should have a policy of reviewing such orders on a regular basis. Any DNAR order only applies to that particular admission for the patient and needs to be renewed on subsequent admissions if still appropriate. It is essential that the medical and nursing staff discuss any decision not to attempt to resuscitate a patient. Any such order should be clearly documented in the nursing notes. In the absence of a DNAR order cardiopulmonary resuscitation must be commenced on every patient irrespective of disease or age. Guidelines on the application of such policies have been published jointly by the British Medical Association, the Royal College of Nursing, and the Resuscitation Council (UK).

Medical emergency teams

It has been recognised for some time that many patients in hospital show clinical signs and symptoms that herald an imminent cardiac and respiratory arrest. These patients have obviously been deteriorating for several hours before they suffer a cardiac arrest. Hospitals are now introducing medical emergency teams to attend to such cases consisting of doctors and nurses experienced in critical care medicine. Specific criteria have been developed to guide ward staff when to call such teams and their introduction has been shown to reduce the incidence of cardiac arrest. Whether survival to hospital discharge is improved is still debatable. The introduction of such teams into hospitals is to be encouraged. Because of the national shortage of "high dependency" beds, some hospitals have critical care nurses to monitor the progress of patients recently discharged from the intensive care unit to a general ward. They watch for any deterioration subsequent to the very significant "step down" in the level of care and expertise that can be provided.

Heartstart UK and community training schemes

All hospitals should encourage community training in basic life support in their catchment area. The hospital management should be encouraged to provide facilities for the community to undertake training within the hospital, using hospital staff and equipment. Schemes such as "Heartstart UK" should be supported and the relatives of patients with cardiac disease and those at high risk of sudden cardiac arrest should be targeted for training

---

Further reading

- Resuscitation Council (UK).*Cardiopulmonary Resuscitation Guidance for Clinical Practice and training in Hospitals.* London: Resuscitation Council (UK), 2000.
- Chamberlain DA, Cummins RO, Abramson N, Allen M. Recommended guidelines for uniform reporting of data from out-of-hospital cardiac arrest: the "Utstein style". *Resuscitation* 1991;22:1-26.
- Royal College of Nursing, British Medical Association. *Cardiopulmonary resuscitation.* London: RCN, 1993.
- Royal College of Physicians. Resuscitation from cardiopulmonary arrest: training and organization. *J R Coll Physicians Lond* 1987;21:1-8.
- Soar J, McKay U. A revised role for the cardiac arrest team? *Resuscitation* 1998;38:145-9.
- Tunstall-Pedoe H, Bailey L, Chamberlain DA, Marsden AK, Ward ME, Zideman DA. Survey of 3765 cardiopulmonary resuscitations in British Hospitals (the BRESUS study): methods and overall results. *BMJ* 1992;304:1347-51.
- Williams R. The "do not resuscitate" decision: guidelines for policy in the adult. *J R Coll Physicians Lond* 1993;27:139-40.

13 Cardiopulmonary resuscitation in primary care

Michael Colquhoun, Brian Steggles

More attempts are now being made in the community to resuscitate patients who suffer cardiopulmonary arrest. In many cases general practitioners and other members of the primary healthcare team will play a vital part, either by initiating treatment themselves or by working with the ambulance service. Few medical emergencies challenge the skills of a medical professional to the same extent as cardiac arrest, and the ability or otherwise of personnel to deal adequately with this situation may literally mean the difference between life and death for the patient.

The public expects doctors, nurses, and members of related professions to be able to manage such emergencies. Studies of resuscitation skills in healthcare professionals have consistently shown major deficiencies in all groups tested. Surveys of those who work in the community have shown that many are inadequately trained to resuscitate patients.

Cardiopulmonary arrest may be a rare event in everyday general practice but it is essential that all members of the primary care team are competent in basic life support and be able to provide immediate treatment (particularly basic life support) for those who collapse with a life-threatening condition.

It is equally important to be able to recognise patients with acute medical conditions that may lead to cardiac arrest because appropriate treatment may prevent its occurrence or increase the chance of full recovery.

Training is not onerous and the equipment required is not excessive compared with the value of a life saved.

Causes of cardiopulmonary arrest

The British Heart Foundation statistics indicate that acute myocardial infarction is the cause of cardiac arrest in 70% of patients in whom resuscitation is attempted by general practitioners, and in the majority of the remaining patients severe coronary disease without actual infarction is responsible for the cardiac arrest. In only 12% of patients is cardiac arrest caused by non-cardiac disease. Other disorders, including valve disease, cardiomyopathy, aortic aneurysm, cerebrovascular disease, and subarachnoid haemorrhage, are among some of the vascular causes of cardiac arrest treated by general practitioners. Non-vascular causes include trauma, electrocution, respiratory disease, near drowning, intoxication, hypovolaemia, and drug overdose. In many of these conditions, appropriate management (particularly of the airway) by someone trained in resuscitation skills may prevent cardiac arrest.

Acute myocardial infarction

The statistics given above show how important it is that general practitioners be trained in resuscitation skills; it is not sound practice to attend a case of acute myocardial infarction without being equipped to defibrillate. All front-line ambulances in the United Kingdom now carry a defibrillator, so if the general

---

Recommended equipment for general practice

Basic
- Automated external defibrillator (AED)
- Defibrillator electrodes
- Manual defibrillator
- Pocket mask
- Oxygen cylinders
- Hand-held suction device

For use by trained staff
- Oropharyngeal or Guedel airway
- Laerdal mask airway

Drugs
- Adrenaline (epinephrine)
- Atropine
- Amiodarone
- Naloxone

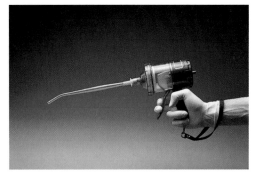

A hand operated pump is one of the pieces of equipment recommended for general practice

Coronary heart disease is the commonest cause of sudden cardiac death, and cardiac arrest is particularly likely to occur in the early stages of myocardial infarction. About two thirds of all patients who die of coronary disease do so outside hospital, around half in the first hour after the onset of symptoms because of the development of ventricular fibrillation. This lethal, yet readily treatable, arrhythmia (sometimes preceded by ventricular tachycardia) is responsible for 85-90% of cases of sudden death

practitioner does not have access to one, he or she should attend with the ambulance service. Such a dual response is recommended for the management of myocardial infarction and has several advantages. The general practitioner will be aware of the patient's history and can provide diagnostic skills, administer opioid analgesics, and treat left ventricular failure while the ambulance service can provide the defibrillator and skilled help should cardiac arrest occur. Some practitioners will also administer thrombolytic drugs to patients with acute myocardial infarction and achieve a worthwhile saving in "pain to needle" time. When a call is received that a patient has collapsed, the same dual response should be instigated.

Practice organisation

Staff who receive emergency calls must be aware of the importance of symptoms like collapse or chest pain and pass the call on to the doctor without delay.

Cardiac arrest may occur on the surgery premises when no doctor is immediately available. All reception and secretarial staff should, therefore, be competent in the techniques of basic life support with the use of a pocket mask or similar device; these techniques should be practised regularly on a training manikin. Practice Nurses and District Nurses should be expert in performing basic life support and, when a practice owns a defibrillator, they should be trained and competent in its use. Such trained nurses may also provide valuable assistance on an emergency call. It is possible that the advent of the first responder automated external defibrillator (AED) (see Chapter 3) will bring defibrillation within the scope of reception and other ancillary staff interested in first aid.

All personnel who provide care for patients with acute myocardial infarction should be equipped and trained to deal with the most common lethal complication of acute coronary syndromes; 5% of all patients with acute infarction attended by a general practitioner experience a cardiac arrest in his or her presence. In one published series the presenting rhythm was one likely to respond to a DC shock in 90% of patients; 75% of patients were initially resuscitated and admitted to hospital alive and 63% were discharged alive.

Resuscitation equipment

Resuscitation equipment will be used relatively infrequently and it is preferable to select items that are easy both to use and maintain. Staff must know where to find the equipment when it is needed and need to be trained in its use to a level that is appropriate to the individuals' expected roles. Each practice should have a named person responsible for checking the state of readiness of all resuscitation drugs and equipment, including the AED, on a regular basis. Disposable items, such as adhesive defibrillator electrodes, have a finite shelf life and will require replacement from time to time if unused.

Defibrillators
The principles of defibrillation and the types of defibrillator available are discussed in Chapters 2 and 3. AEDs offer several potential advantages over other methods of defibrillation: the machines are cheaper, smaller, and lighter to carry than conventional defibrillators and they are designed for infrequent use or occasional use with minimal maintenance. Skill in the

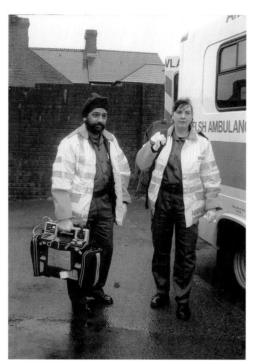

If a general practitioner does not have access to a defibrillator they should attend a case of acute myocardial infarction with the ambulance service

Emergency calls are usually received by receptionists, although other procedures may apply outside office hours. Increasingly, emergency cover is provided by cooperatives or primary care centres based at community hospitals or specially designated premises.

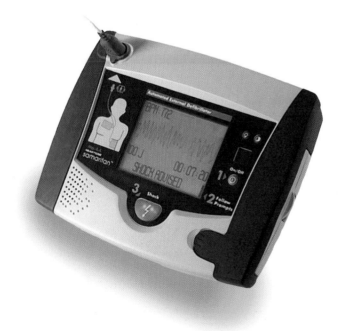

Automated external defibrillator

recognition of electrocardiogram rhythms is not required and the automation of several stages in the process of defibrillation is a distinct advantage to the doctor, who may well be working with very limited help. AEDs have been successfully employed both by general practitioners and lay first aiders in the treatment of patients with ventricular fibrillation in the community.

Airway management

The ability to give expired air ventilation, using a pocket mask with a one way valve, is the minimum skill expected. Other simple airway barrier devices are not as effective as a pocket mask and may provide substantial resistance to lung inflation. Devices such as the oropharyngeal or Guedel airway are suitable for use by those who are appropriately trained; a range of sizes may need to be kept available. For those with appropriate experience, the laryngeal mask airway has an increasing role in the management of the airway in unconscious patients outside hospital. Tracheal intubation and the use of other advanced airway techniques are only appropriate for use by those who have undergone extensive training and who practise the skills regularly.

Training in resuscitation techniques

Training and practice are necessary to acquire skill in resuscitation techniques, and the principles behind such training are covered in Chapter 19. Repeated tuition and practice are the most successful methods of learning and retaining resuscitation skills. The levels of skill required by different members of the primary healthcare team will vary according to the individual's role and, in some cases, their enthusiasm. The aim of an individual healthcare practice should be to provide as competent a response as possible within the resources available.

All those in direct contact with patients should be trained in basic life support and related resuscitation skills, such as the recovery position. As a minimum requirement they should be able to provide effective basic life support with an airway adjunct such as a pocket mask. Doctors, nurses, and healthcare workers, such as physiotherapists, should also be able to use an AED effectively. Other personnel—for example, receptionists— may also be trained to use an AED; they are nearly always present when a practice is open and may have to respond before more highly trained help is available.

Training should be provided for each trainee up to the appropriate level required by their role within the practice. In many cases, particularly for higher levels of skill, the services of a resuscitation officer (RO) will be required. The organisations that manage the provision of primary care (Primary Care Groups or Trusts, Local Healthcare Cooperatives, or Local Health Groups) should consider engaging the services of an RO. Ambulance Service Training Schools can also provide training to a similar level of competency. The Voluntary Aid Societies and comparable organisations train their members in resuscitation skills, including the use of an AED, and may be engaged to provide training for some members of the primary healthcare team. Knowledgeable members of the practice team can undertake training for the other members of their own practice. No evidence base exists on which to make definite recommendations about the frequency of refresher training specifically for those working in primary healthcare teams. The consensus view, based on studies of comparable providers, suggests that doctors and nurses should have refresher training in basic life support every six to 12 months. Retraining in the

> Manual defibrillators may be appropriate for use in general practice, but the greater training required and the fact that they are less portable limits the number of staff who can use them

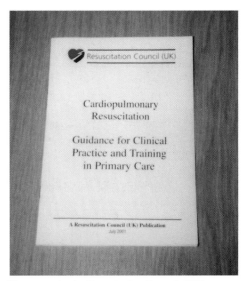

The report by the Resuscitation Council (UK) entitled *Cardiopulmonary Resuscitation Guidance for Clinical Practice and Training in Primary Care* recommends that all practices should acquire an AED and that they should be available to those providing cover out-of-hours, whether it be in a primary care centre or as part of a deputising service or cooperative.

Oxygen

Current resuscitation guidelines emphasise the use of oxygen, and this should be available whenever possible. Oxygen cylinders should be appropriately maintained and the national safety standards followed. Every practice should have guidelines that allow non-medical staff to administer high-flow oxygen

Suction

The requirement for batteries is a disadvantage for suction equipment that is likely to be used infrequently. Similarly, the need for mains electricity adds greatly to the cost and restricts the location where a suction device can be used. For these reasons, simple mechanical portable hand-held suction devices are recommended

Drugs

The role of drugs in the management of cardiopulmonary arrest is discussed in detail in Chapter 16. No drug has been shown convincingly to influence the outcome of cardiopulmonary arrest, and few are therefore recommended for routine use

Universal precautions

Standard procedures should be followed to minimise the risk of cross infection. Gloves should be available together with a suitable means of disposing of contaminated sharps

use of the AED for this group of workers should be carried out at least as often.

The importance of acquiring and maintaining competency in resuscitation skills may be an appropriate subject to include in an employee's job description. It is also a suitable subject for inclusion in individual personal development plans and may in due course form part of re-validation procedures.

Ethical issues

It is essential to identify individuals in whom cardiopulmonary arrest is a terminal event and when resuscitation is inappropriate. Community hospitals, hospices, nursing homes, and similar establishments where the primary healthcare team is responsible for the care of patients should be encouraged to implement "do not attempt resuscitation" (DNAR) policies so that inappropriate or unwanted resuscitation attempts are avoided. National guidelines published by the British Medical Association, the Resuscitation Council (UK), and the Royal College of Nursing provide detailed guidance on which local practice can be based.

The overall responsibility for a DNAR decision in the community rests with the doctor in charge of the patient's care, which will usually be the general practitioner. The opinions of other members of the medical and nursing team, the patient, and their relatives should be taken into account in reaching the decision. The most senior member of the medical team should enter the DNAR decision and the reason for it in the medical records. Exactly what relatives have been told should be documented, together with any additional comments made at the time. This decision should be reviewed regularly in the light of the patient's condition. Any such DNAR decision should also be recorded in the nursing notes when applicable and be effectively communicated to all members of the multi-disciplinary team involved in the patient's care. This should include all those who may become involved, such as the emergency medical services, so that inappropriate 999 telephone calls at the time of death are avoided.

Performance management

The procedures carried out and the outcome of all resuscitation attempts should be the subject of audit. This may be carried out either by an individual practice or at a local level in which a number of practices provide the primary care service.

A local review of resuscitation attempts should highlight serious deficiencies in training, equipment, or procedures. The Risk Manager of a primary care organisation should be made aware of any problems, difficulties, or considerations of relevance in the locality in which they serve. When an audit has identified deficiencies, it is imperative that steps are taken to improve performance. The training received by members of the primary healthcare team is also a suitable subject for audit and might be undertaken at both practice level or within the primary care organisation.

Accurate records of all resuscitation attempts should be kept for audit, training, and medical legal reasons. The responsibility for this will rest with the most senior member of the practice team. Such records may need to be sent to the Risk Manager or Record Management Department of the local primary care organisation. The electronic data stored by most AEDs during a resuscitation attempt is an additional resource that should be used for audit purposes. The effectiveness of local DNAR policies is also a suitable subject for audit.

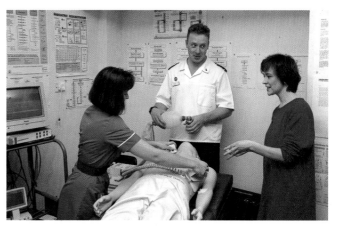

Refresher training Courses are important for those in primary health care teams

Recommended training and practice for primary care staff in contact with patients

Basic
- Basic life support
- Use of airway adjunct such as pocket mask
- Use of AED

Advanced
- Intravenous access and infusion
- Analgesia for patients with myocardial infarction
- Rhythm recognition and treatment of peri-arrest arrhythmias
- Advanced airway management techniques
- Use of drugs
- Principles of management of trauma

Training
- Training to appropriate level
- Resuscitation officer training for higher skills
- Regular training update, preferably every six months

The audit should include the availability and performance of individuals involved in the resuscitation attempts and the standard, availability, and reliability of the equipment used. The methods by which urgent calls are received and processed should be the subject of regular review and is also a suitable subject for audit at practice level. This could take the form of critical incident debriefing

Useful addresses
- The Faculty of Pre-hospital Care. The Royal College of Surgeons of Edinburgh, Nicolson Street, Edinburgh EH8 9DW. Tel: 0131 527 1600
- British Association for Immediate Medical Care (BASICS), Turret House, Turret Lane, Ipswich IP4 1DL. Tel: 0870 16549999
- British Heart Foundation, 14 Fitzhardinge Street, London W1H 6DH. Tel: 020 7935 0185

Pre-hospital care

For many years suitably trained and equipped doctors in the United Kingdom, principally general practitioners, have worked with the emergency services to provide medical assistance and to resuscitate patients who have had accidents or serious medical emergencies. Many such local immediate care schemes belong to the British Association for Immediate Care. The Faculty of Pre-hospital Care was established by the Royal College of Surgeons of Edinburgh in 1996, with the principal aim of embracing all activity in the field of pre-hospital care and the professions involved in that work. The faculty is actively involved in training for those who provide pre-hospital care and holds both Diploma and Fellowship examinations in Immediate Medical Care.

Further reading

- Resuscitation Council (UK). *Cardiopulmonary resuscitation: guidance for clinical practice and training in primary care.* London: Resuscitation Council (UK), 2001.
- Colquhoun MC. Defibrillation by general practitioners. *Resuscitation* 2002;52:143-8.
- Colquhoun MC, Jevon P. *Resuscitation in primary care.* Oxford: Butterworth Heinemann, 2001.
- Pai GR, Naites NE, Rawles JM. One thousand heart attacks in the Grampion. The place of cardiopulmonary resuscitation in general practice. *BMJ* 1987;294:352-4.
- British Medical Association Resuscitation Council (UK), Royal College of Nursing. Decisions relating to cardiopulmonary resuscitation. A joint statement from the British Medical Association, The Resuscitation Council (UK) and the Royal College of Nursing. London: British Medical Association, 2001.
- Weston CFM, Penny WJ, Julian DG. On behalf of the British Heart Foundation Working Group. Guidelines for the early management of patients with myocardial infarction. *BMJ* 1994;308:767-71.

14 Resuscitation of the patient with major trauma

Charles D Deakin

In the United Kingdom, trauma is the most common cause of death in patients aged below 40 years, accounting for over 3000 deaths and 30 000 serious injuries each year. The landmark report of the Royal College of Surgeons (1988) on the management of patients with major injuries highlighted serious deficiencies in trauma management in the United Kingdom. In the same year, the introduction of the American College of Surgeon's Advanced Trauma Life Support course aimed to improve standards of trauma care, emphasising the importance of a structured approach to treatment.

Resuscitation of the trauma patient entails a primary survey followed by a secondary survey. The primary survey aims to identify and treat life-threatening conditions immediately and follows the well established sequence of A (airway and cervical spine stabilisation), B (breathing), C (circulation), D [disability (neurological assessment)], and E (exposure). The secondary survey is based on an anatomical examination of the head, chest, abdomen, genito-urinary system, limbs, and back and aims to provide a thorough check of the entire body. Any sudden deterioration or adverse change in the patient's condition during this approach necessitates repeating the primary survey to identify new life-threatening conditions.

Management and treatment of cardiac arrest in trauma patients follows the principles detailed in earlier chapters. The primary arrhythmia in adult traumatic cardiac arrest is pulseless electrical activity (PEA), and specific causes should be sought and treated. Paediatric traumatic arrests are usually due to hypoxia or neurological injury, but, in either case, adequate ventilation is particularly important in the management of these patients.

Receiving the patient

Management of the trauma patient in hospital should begin with a clear and concise handover from the ambulance crew, who should give a summary of the incident, the mechanism of injury, the clinical condition of the patient on scene, suspected injuries, and any treatment given in the pre-hospital setting. During this handover, it is imperative that the receiving team remain silent and listen to these important details.

Trauma team

It is important that a well organised trauma team should receive the patient. Ideally this will comprise a team leader, an "airway" doctor, and two "circulation" doctors, each doctor being paired with a member of the nursing team. An additional nurse may be designated to care for relatives; a radiographer forms the final team member.

Primary survey

Airway and cervical spine stabilisation

Airway
Some degree of airway obstruction is the rule rather than the exception in patients with major trauma and is present in as

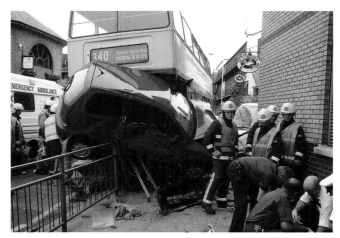

In the United Kingdom, trauma is the most common cause of death in patients aged less than 40 years

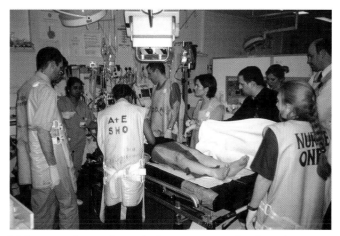

It is important that a well organised trauma team receives the patient

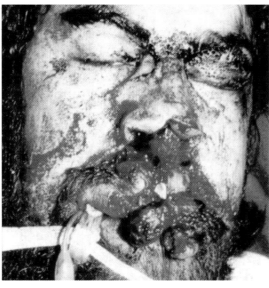

The airway is at risk from blood, tissue debris, swelling, vomit, and mechanical disruption

many as 85% of patients who have "survivable" injuries but nevertheless die after major trauma. The aim of airway management is to allow both adequate oxygenation to prevent tissue hypoxia and adequate ventilation to prevent hypercapnia.

The airway is at risk from:

- Blood
- Tissue debris
- Swelling
- Vomit
- Mechanical disruption.

Loss of consciousness diminishes the protective upper airway reflexes (cough and gag), endangering the airway further through aspiration and its sequelae.

Examine the patient for airway obstruction. If the patient is able to talk it means that the airway is patent and breathing and the circulation is adequate to perfuse the brain with oxygenated blood. Signs of airway obstruction include:

- Stridor (may be absent in complete obstruction)
- Cyanosis
- Tracheal tug
- "See-saw" respiration
- Inadequate chest wall movement.

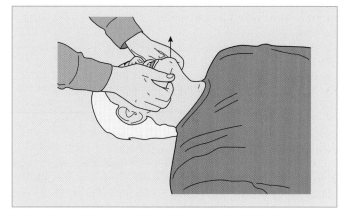

Jaw thrust opens the airway while maintaining cervical spine alignment

Oxygen

Aim to give 100% oxygen to all patients by delivering 15 l/min through an integrated mask and reservoir bag. Lower concentrations of oxygen should not be given to trauma patients with chronic obstructive pulmonary disease even though they may rely on hypoxic drive. However, respiratory deterioration in these patients will necessitate intubation.

Basic airway manoeuvres

Manoeuvres to open the airway differ from those used in the management of primary cardiac arrest. The standard head tilt and chin lift results in significant extension of the cervical spine and is inappropriate when cervical spine injury is suspected. Airway manoeuvres must keep the cervical spine in a neutral alignment. These are:

- Jaw thrust—the rescuer's fingers are placed along the angle of the jaw with the thumbs placed on the maxilla. The jaw is then lifted, drawing it anteriorly, thus opening the airway
- Chin lift—this achieves the same as a jaw thrust by lifting the tip of the jaw anteriorly.

Airway adjuncts

If basic airway manoeuvres fail to clear the airway, consider the use of adjuncts, such as an oropharyngeal (Guedel) or nasopharyngeal airway. The oropharyngeal airway is inserted into the mouth inverted and then rotated 180° before being inserted fully over the tongue. The nasopharyngeal airway is inserted backwards into the nostril as far as the proximal flange, using a safety pin to prevent it slipping into the nostril. It should be used with caution in patients with suspected basal skull fracture.

Suction is an important adjunct to airway management. Blood, saliva, and vomit frequently contribute to airway obstruction and must be removed promptly. Be careful not to trigger vomiting in patients who are semi-conscious. Be prepared to roll the patient and tip them head down if they vomit, taking particular care of those who cannot protect their airway—for example, those who are unconscious or those on a spinal board.

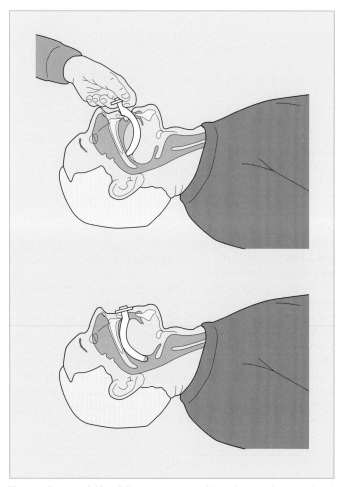

The oropharyngeal (Guedel) airway is inserted into the mouth inverted and then rotated 180° before being inserted fully over the tongue

Definitive airways

It is important to secure the airway early to allow effective ventilation. The gold standard is endotracheal intubation because a cuffed tracheal tube isolates the airway from ingress of debris.

Endotracheal intubation is a skill requiring considerable experience and is more difficult in trauma patients. Unless patients are completely obtunded with a Glasgow Coma Score (GCS) of 3, intubation can only be performed safely with the use of anaesthetic drugs and neuromuscular blocking drugs, together with cricoid pressure to prevent aspiration of gastric contents.

Distorted anatomy, blood, and secretions, and the presence of a hard cervical collar all impair visualisation of the vocal cords. Removal of the collar and use of manual inline stabilisation will improve the view at laryngoscopy. Better visualisation of the vocal cords may be obtained by using the flexible tip of a McCoy laryngoscope, and cricoid pressure, directed backwards, upwards, and to the right (BURP manoeuvre), may also improve visualisation.

A gum elastic bougie, with a tracheal tube "railroaded" over it, can be used to intubate the cords when they are not directly visible. Once the tracheal tube is inserted it is vital to confirm that it is in the correct position, particularly to exclude oesophageal intubation. Look and listen (with a stethoscope) for equal chest movement, and listen over the epigastrium to exclude air entry in the stomach, which occurs after oesophageal intubation. Capnography (measurement of expired carbon dioxide) is the best method of confirming tracheal placement, either using direct measurement of exhaled gases or watching for the change of colour of carbon dioxide sensitive paper.

The laryngeal mask airway (LMA) and Combi-tube have both been advocated as alternative airways when endotracheal intubation fails or is not possible. The LMA is relatively easy to insert and does not require visualisation of the vocal cords for insertion. The cuff forms a loose seal over the laryngeal inlet but only provides limited protection of the trachea from aspiration. The Combi-tube is also inserted blind. It is a double lumen tube, the tip of which may either enter the trachea or, more usually, the oesophagus. Once inserted, the operator has to identify the position of the tube and ventilate the patient using the appropriate lumen. Neither of these devices should be used by operators unfamiliar with their insertion.

Surgical airway
A surgical approach is necessary if other means of securing a clear airway fail. Access is gained to the trachea through the cricothyroid membrane and overlying skin. Several techniques are used as described below.

Needle cricothyroidotomy—a large (14G +) needle is inserted through the cricothyroid membrane in the midline. Spontaneous respiration is not possible through such a small lumen and high-pressure oxygen must be delivered down the cannula. A three-way tap or the side-port of a "Y" connector allows intermittent insufflation (one second on, four seconds off). This technique delivers adequate oxygen but fails to clear carbon dioxide and can only be used for periods not exceeding 30 minutes. Care must be taken to ensure that airway obstruction does not prevent insufflated air from escaping through the laryngeal inlet.

Insertion of "minitrach" device—the "minitrach" has become popular as a device for obtaining a surgical airway. It is a short, 4.0 mm, uncuffed tube that is inserted through the cricothyroid membrane using a Seldinger technique. A guidewire is inserted through a hollow needle, the needle removed and the minitrach introduced over the guidewire. It is too small to allow spontaneous ventilation, but oxygen can be delivered as with a needle cricothyroidotomy or using a self-inflating ventilation bag.

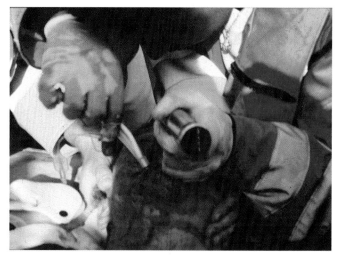

Removal of the hard collar and use of manual inline stabilisation will improve the view at laryngoscopy

---

Indications for endotracheal intubation are:

- Apnoea
- Failure of basic airway manoeuvres to maintain an airway
- Failure to maintain adequate oxygenation via a face mask
- Protection of the airway from blood or vomit
- Head injury requiring ventilation
- Progressive airway swelling likely to cause obstruction—for example, upper airway burns.

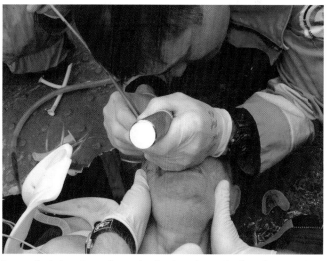

A gum elastic bougie can be used to intubate the cords when they are not directly visible

Surgical cricothyroidotomy—surgical cricothyroidotomy is the most difficult of the three procedures to perform but provides the best airway. A large, preferably transverse, incision is made in the cricothyroid membrane through both overlying the skin and the membrane itself. Tracheal dilators are then used to expand the incision and a cuffed tracheostomy tube (6.0-8.0 mm) is inserted into the trachea. An alternative technique entails insertion of a gum elastic bougie through the incision with a 6.0 mm cuffed endotracheal tube "railroaded" over it. Care must be taken not to advance the tube into the right main bronchus.

Cervical spine

An injury to the cervical spine occurs in about 5% of patients who suffer blunt trauma, whereas the incidence with penetrating trauma is less than 1%, provided that the neck is not directly involved. It is important to assume that all patients with major trauma have an unstable cervical spine injury until proven otherwise.

Cervical spine stabilisation should be carried out at the same time as airway management. Most patients with suspected cervical spine injuries will be delivered by the ambulance crew on a spinal board with a hard collar, head blocks, and straps already in place. If not, manual inline stabilisation must be applied immediately, and a hard collar fitted, together with lateral support and tape. Some compromise may be necessary if the patient is uncooperative because attempts to fit a hard collar may cause excessive cervical spine movement.

Hard collars must be fitted correctly; too short a collar will provide inadequate support, whereas too tall a collar may hyperextend the neck. The collar must be reasonably tight, otherwise the chin tends to slip below the chin support. Several different types of hard collar are available. One commonly used is the Stifneck™ extrication collar, which is sized by measuring the vertical distance from the top of the patient's shoulders to the bottom of the chin with the head in a neutral position. Sizing posts on the collar are then adjusted to the same distance before the collar is fitted to the patient.

Once the head is secured firmly in head blocks, consider loosening or removing the cervical collar because evidence shows that tight collars can cause an increase in intracranial pressure. Pressure sores are also a risk if the hard collar is left in place for several days. Patients should also be removed from the spinal board as soon as possible.

Breathing

Once the airway has been secured, attention must be turned to assessment of breathing and identification of any life-threatening conditions. The chest must be exposed and examined carefully. Assess the respiratory rate and effort and examine for symmetry of chest excursion. Look for any signs of injury, such as entry wounds of penetrating trauma or bruising from blunt trauma. Feel for surgical emphysema, which is often associated with rib fractures, a pneumothorax, flail segment, or upper airway disruption.

Five main life-threatening thoracic conditions that must be identified and treated immediately are:

- Tension pneumothorax
- Haemothorax
- Flail chest
- Cardiac tamponade
- Open chest wound.

Tension pneumothorax causes respiratory and circulatory collapse within minutes and is often exacerbated by positive pressure ventilation. Asymmetric chest wall excursion,

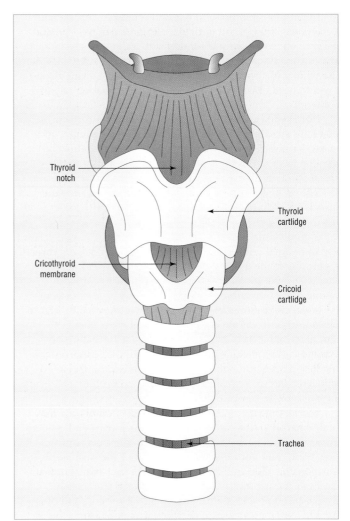

Anatomical location of the cricothyroid membrane

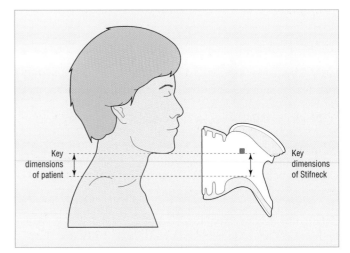

Sizing of the "Stifneck" collar

If all the following criteria are met, cervical spine stabilisation is unnecessary:

- No neck pain
- No localised tenderness
- No neurological signs or symptoms
- No loss of consciousness
- No distracting injury
- Patient alert and oriented

contralateral tracheal deviation, absent breath sounds, and hyperresonance to percussion all indicate a significant tension pneumothorax. Initial treatment by needle decompression aims to relieve pressure quickly before insertion of a definitive chest drain. Needle decompression is performed by inserting a 14G cannula through the second intercostal space (immediately above the top of the third rib) in the midclavicular line. In the 5% of patients who have a chest wall thickness greater than 4.5 cm, a longer needle or rapid insertion of a chest drain is required.

Haemothorax is suggested by absent breath sounds and stony dullness to percussion. The presence of air (haemopneumothorax) may mask dullness to percussion, particularly in a supine patient. It requires prompt insertion of a chest drain. Bleeding at more than 200 ml/hour may require surgical intervention.

Flail chest occurs when multiple rib fractures result in a free segment of chest wall that moves paradoxically with respiration. Patients are at risk of both haemothorax and pneumothorax and will rapidly progress to respiratory failure. Early endotracheal intubation is required.

Not all these features may be present in clinical practice. Heart sounds are often quiet in hypovolaemic patients and central venous pressure may not be raised if the patient is hypovolaemic. Pericardiocentesis is performed by insertion of a needle 1-2 cm inferior to the left xiphochondral junction with a wide bore cannula aimed laterally and posteriorly at 45° towards the tip of the left scapula. Connecting an electrocardiogram (ECG) to the needle and observing for injury potential as the needle penetrates the myocardium has traditionally been advocated as a means of confirming anatomical location. Nowadays, many accident and emergency departments have access to portable ultrasound, which provides better visualisation.

Open chest wounds require covering with a three-sided dressing (to prevent formation of a tension pneumothorax) or an Asherman seal together with early insertion of a chest drain.

Blunt trauma is associated with pulmonary contusion, which may not be apparent on early chest x ray examination but can result in significantly impaired gas exchange.

Circulation

Hypovolaemic shock is a state in which oxygen delivery to the tissues fails to match oxygen demand. It rapidly leads to tissue hypoxia, anaerobic metabolism, cellular injury, and irreversible damage to vital organs. Although external haemorrhage is obvious, occult bleeding into body cavities is common and the chest, abdomen, and pelvis must be examined carefully in hypovolaemic patients. Isolated head injuries rarely cause hypotension (although blood loss from scalp lacerations can be significant).

Estimation of blood loss, particularly on scene, is inaccurate but nevertheless provides some indication of the severity of external haemorrhage. Assessment of the circulatory system begins with a clinical examination of the pulse, blood pressure, capillary refill time, pallor, peripheral circulation, and level of consciousness. Most physiological variables in adults change little until more than 30% blood volume has been lost; children compensate even more effectively. Any patient who is hypotensive through blood loss has, therefore, lost a significant volume and further loss may result in haemodynamic collapse.

Hypovolaemic shock has been classified into four broad classes (I-IV).

- Class I is blood loss less than 15% total blood volume (750 ml) during which physiological variables change little
- Class II is blood loss of 15-30% (800-1500 ml), which results in a moderate tachycardia and delayed capillary refill but no change in systolic blood pressure

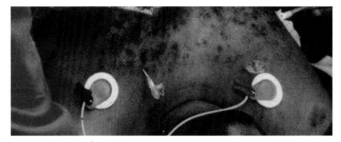

Bilateral needle decompression (note that the left-sided needle has become dislodged)

Cardiac tamponade is diagnosed by the classic Beck's triad:

- Muffled heart sounds
- Raised central venous pressure
- Systemic hypotension

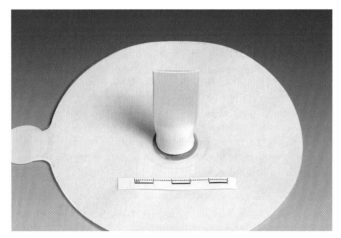

Asherman seal

Classification of hypovolaemic shock and changes in physiological variables

	Class I	Class II	Class III	Class IV
Blood loss				
%	<15	15-30	30-40	>40
ml	750	800-1500	1500-2000	2000
Blood pressure				Very low
Systolic	Normal	Normal	Decreased	Barely
Diastolic	Normal	Decreased	Decreased	recordable
Pulse (beats/min)	Normal	100-120	120 (thready)	120 (very thready)
Capillary refill	Normal	Slow (>2 seconds)	Slow (>2 seconds)	Undetectable
Respiratory rate	Normal	Tachypnoea	Tachypnoea (>20/min)	Tachypnoea (20/min)
Extremities	Normal	Pale	Pale	Clammy, cold
Mental state	Alert	Restless or aggressive	Anxious, drowsy, aggressive	Drowsy, confused or unconscious

- Class III is blood loss of 30-40% (1500-2000 ml), which is associated with a thready tachycardic pulse, systolic hypotension, pallor, and delayed capillary refill
- Class IV blood loss is in excess of 45% (more than 2000 ml) and is associated with barely detectable pulses, extreme hypotension, and a reduced level of consciousness
- Some texts claim that the radial, femoral, and carotid pulses disappear sequentially as blood pressure falls below specific levels. This technique tends to overestimate blood pressure; the radial pulse may still be palpable at pressures considerably lower than a systolic of 80 mmHg.

Blood tests are of little use in the initial assessment of haemorrhage because the haematocrit is unchanged immediately after an acute bleed.

Management of haemorrhage

External bleeding can often be controlled by firm compression and elevation. Compression of a major vessel (for example, femoral artery) may be more effective than compression over the wound itself. Internal bleeding requires immediate surgical haemostasis.

Intravenous access

Two large-bore intravenous cannulae (14G+) should be inserted. These can be used to draw blood samples for cross-match, full blood count, urea, and electrolytes. Central venous access allows measurement of central venous pressure as a means of judging the adequacy of volume expansion. It should only be undertaken by an experienced physician because the procedure may be difficult in a hypovolaemic patient. Recent guidelines from the National Institute for Clinical Excellence recommend using ultrasound to locate the vein. After insertion, a chest x ray examination is necessary to exclude an iatrogenic pneumothorax.

Over the past decade, management of hypovolaemic shock has moved away from restoration of blood volume to a normovolaemic state to one of permissive hypotension. Blood volume is restored only to levels that allow vital organ perfusion (heart, brain) without accelerating blood loss, which is generally considered to be a systolic blood pressure of about 80 mmHg. Permissive hypotension has been shown to improve morbidity and mortality in animal models and clinical studies of acute hypovolaemia secondary to penetrating trauma. The benefits of permissive hypotension may also apply to haemorrhage secondary to blunt trauma.

Patients with raised intracranial pressure may need higher blood pressures to maintain adequate cerebral perfusion. The same may be true for trauma patients with chronic hypertension.

Debate still continues as to the optimal fluid for resuscitation in acute hypovolaemia. It is the volume of fluid that is probably the most important factor in initial resuscitation. As a general rule, isotonic saline (0.9%) is a suitable fluid with which to commence volume resuscitation. After the initial 2000 ml of 0.9% saline, colloid may be considered if further volume expansion is required. Once 30-40% blood volume has been replaced, it is necessary to consider the additional use of blood. Intravenous fluid resuscitation in children should begin with boluses of 20 ml/kg, titrated according to effect.

Crystalloids

Crystalloids freely cross capillary membranes and equilibrate within the whole intracellular and extracellular fluid spaces. As a result, intravascular retention of crystalloids is poor

In patients with impalpable pulses, the causes of PEA must be actively sought and excluded:

- Hypovolaemia
- Hypothermia
- Hypoxaemia
- Tamponade (cardiac)
- Tension pneumothorax
- Acidosis

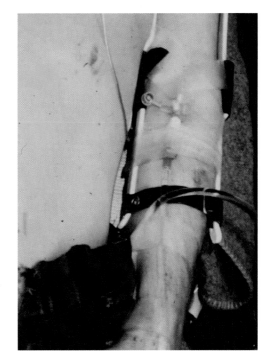

Intravenous access

Excess intravenous fluid given before surgical haemostasis is achieved may have a detrimental effect for several reasons:

- Increased blood pressure dislodges blood clots
- Increased blood pressure accelerates bleeding
- Bleeding requires further fluids, resulting in a dilutional coagulopathy
- Intravenous fluids generally cause hypothermia
- Hypothermia may result in arrhythmias

(about 20%) and at least three times the actual intravascular volume deficit must be infused to achieve normovolaemia.

Colloids

Colloids are large molecules that remain in the intravascular compartment until they are metabolised. Therefore, they provide more efficient volume restoration than crystalloids. After one to two hours, the plasma volume supporting effect is similar to that seen with crystalloids. The main colloids available are derived from gelatins:

- Gelofusine
- Haemaccel (unsuitable for transfusion with whole blood because of its high calcium content).

Hypertonic saline

Hypertonic saline (7.5%) is an effective volume expander, the effects of which are prolonged if combined with the hydrophilic effects of dextran 70. In an adult, about 250 ml (4 ml/kg) hypertonic saline dextran (HSD) provides a similar haemodynamic response to that seen with 3000 ml of 0.9% normal saline. Hypertonic saline acts through several pathways to improve hypovolaemic shock:

- Effective intravascular volume expansion and improved organ blood flow
- Reduced endothelial swelling, improving microcirculatory blood flow
- Lowering of intracranial pressure through an osmotic effect.

Clinical studies are limited but some evidence shows that HSD may be of benefit in patients with head injury in particular.

Blood

Once a patient has lost more than 30-40% of their blood volume, a transfusion will be required to maintain adequate oxygen-carrying capacity. Appropriately cross-matched blood is ideal, but the urgency of the situation may only allow time to complete a type-specific cross-match or necessitate the immediate use of "O" rhesus negative blood. Aim to maintain haemoglobin above 8.0 g/dl. Deranged coagulation may be a significant problem with massive transfusion, requiring administration of clotting products and platelets.

Intravenous fluids should ideally be warmed before administration to minimise hypothermia; 500 ml blood at 4°C will reduce core temperature by about 0.5°C. Large volumes of cold fluids can, therefore, cause significant hypothermia, which is itself associated with significant morbidity and mortality.

If the patient is pregnant the gravid uterus should be displaced laterally to avoid hypotension associated with aortocaval compression; blankets under the right hip will suffice if a wedge is not available. If the patient requires immobilisation on a spinal board, place the wedge underneath the board.

Disability (neurological)

A rapid assessment of neurological status is performed as part of the primary survey. Although an altered level of consciousness may be caused by head injury, hypoxia and hypotension are also common causes of central nervous system depression. Be careful not to attribute a depressed level of consciousness to alcohol in a patient who has been drinking. Regular re-evaluation of disability is essential to monitor trends. A more detailed assessment using the Glasgow Coma Score can be performed with the primary or secondary survey.

Crystalloids

Advantages
- Balanced electrolyte composition
- Buffering capacity (lactate)
- No risk of anaphylaxis
- Little disturbance to haemostasis
- Promotes diuresis
- Cheap

Disadvantages
- Poor plasma volume expansion
- Large quantities needed
- Risk of hypothermia
- Reduced plasma colloid osmotic pressure
- Tissue oedema
- Contributes to multiple organ dysfunction syndrome

Colloids

Advantages
- Effective plasma volume expansion
- Moderately prolonged increase in plasma volume
- Moderate volumes required
- Maintain plasma colloid osmotic pressure
- Minimal risk of tissue oedema

Disadvantages
- Risk of anaphylactoid reactions
- Some disturbance of haemostasis
- Moderately expensive

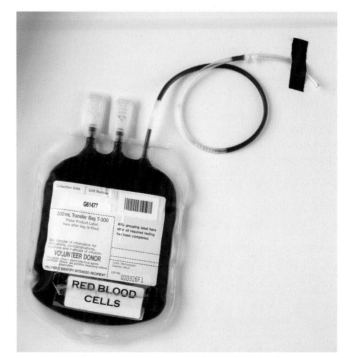

Blood—one unit of packed cells will raise the haemoglobin by about 1 g/l

It is important to document pupillary size and reaction to light. If spinal injury is suspected, cord function (gross motor and sensory evaluation of each limb) should be documented early, preferably before endotracheal intubation. High-dose corticosteroids have been shown to reduce the degree of neurological deficit if given within the first 24 hours after injury. Methylprednisolone is generally recommended, as early as possible: 30 mg/kg intravenously over 15 minutes followed by an infusion of 5.4 mg/kg/hour for 23 hours.

> **Neurological status can be assessed using the simple AVPU mnemonic:**
> - Alert
> - Responds to voice
> - Responds to pain
> - Unconscious

Glasgow Coma Scale

Eye opening		Verbal response		Motor response	
Spontaneously	4	Orientated	5	Obeys commands	6
To speech	3	Confused	4	Localises to pain	5
To pain	2	Inappropriate words	3	Flexion (withdrawal)	4
Never	1	Incomprehensible sounds	2	Flexion (decerebrate)	3
		Silent	1	Extension	2
				No response	1

Exposure

Remove any remaining clothing to allow a complete examination; log roll the patient to examine the back. Hypothermia should be actively prevented by maintaining a warm environment, keeping the patient covered when possible, warming intravenous fluids, and using forced air warming devices.

Secondary survey

The secondary survey commences once the primary survey is complete, and it entails a meticulous head-to-toe evaluation.

Head

Examine the scalp, head, and neck for lacerations, contusions, and evidence of fractures. Examine the eyes before eyelid oedema makes this difficult. Look in the ears for cerebrospinal fluid leaks, tympanic membrane integrity, and to exclude a haemotympanum.

Thorax

Re-examine the chest for signs of bruising, lacerations, deformity, and asymmetry. Arrhythmias or acute ischaemic changes on the ECG may indicate cardiac contusion. A plain chest x ray is important to exclude pneumothorax, haemothorax, and diaphragmatic hernia; a widened mediastinum may indicate aortic injury and requires a chest computerised tomography, which is also useful in the detection of rib fractures that may be missed on a plain chest x ray. Fluid levels in the chest will only be apparent on x ray if the patient is erect.

Abdomen

Examine the abdomen for bruising and swelling. Carefully palpate each of the four quadrants; large volumes of blood can be lost into the abdomen, usually from hepatic or splenic injuries, without gross clinical signs. Diagnostic peritoneal lavage or ultrasonography can be performed quickly in the accident and emergency department. Exploratory laparotomy must be performed urgently when intra-abdominal bleeding is suspected. Women of childbearing age should have a pregnancy test.

> A comatose patient (GCS <8) will require endotracheal intubation. Secondary brain injury is minimised by ensuring adequate oxygenation (patent airway), adequate ventilation (to prevent cerebral vasodilatation caused by hypercapnia), and the treatment of circulatory shock to ensure adequate cerebral perfusion. Prompt neurosurgical review is vital, particularly in patients who have clinical or radiographic evidence of an expanding space-occupying lesion

Summary

- Management of the patient with acute trauma begins with a primary survey aimed at identifying and treating life-threatening injuries. It entails exposing the patient to allow examination of the airway, breathing, circulation, and disability (neurological examination)
- The secondary survey is a thorough head-to-toe examination to assess all injuries and enable a treatment plan to be formulated

Further reading

- American College of Surgeons. *Advanced Trauma Life Support Course*® *Manual.* American College of Surgeons. 6th ed. 1997.
- Alderson P, Schierhout G, Roberts I, Bunn F. Colloids vs crystalloids for fluid resuscitation in critically ill patients. (Cochrane Review). In: *The Cochrane Library,* Issue 3. Oxford: Update Software, 2002.
- Driscoll P, Skinner D, Earlam R. *ABC of Major Trauma.* 3rd ed. London: BMJ Books, 2000.
- National Institute for Clinical Excellence. *Guidance on the use of ultrasound locating devices for placing central venous catheters.* Technology Appraisal Guidance No.49. September 2002. London: NICE, 2002.

Limbs
These should be examined for tenderness, bruising, and deformity. A careful neurological and vascular assessment must be made and any fractures reduced and splinted.

Spinal column
The patient should be log rolled to examine the spine for tenderness and deformity. Sensory and motor deficits, priapism, and reduced anal tone will indicate the level of any cord lesion. Neurogenic shock is manifest by bradycardia and hypotension, the severity of which depends on the cord level of the lesion.

The line drawings in this chapter are adapted from the *ALS Course Provider Manual*. 4th ed. London: Resuscitation Council (UK), 2000. The photograph of the airway at risk is reproduced for the from the chapter on Maxillofacial injuries by Iain Hutchison and Perter Hardee in the *ABC of Major Trauma*. 3rd ed. London: BMJ Publishing Group, 2000.

15 Near drowning

Mark Harries

Introduction

At times, cold can protect life as well as endanger it. There have been extraordinary examples of survival after very long periods of submersion in ice-cold water. Such cases highlight the differences in the approach to resuscitation that sets the management of individuals who nearly drown apart from all other circumstances in which cardiopulmonary arrest has occurred.

Management at the scene

Rewarming

Attempts to rewarm patients with deep hypothermia outside hospital are inappropriate but measures to prevent further heat loss are important. Good evidence suggests that when cardiac arrest has occurred, chest compression alone is as effective as chest compression with expired air resuscitation. Extracorporeal rewarming plays such an important role that unconscious patients with deep hypothermia should not be transported to a hospital that lacks these facilities.

To prevent further heat loss in conscious patients with hypothermia, wet clothing should be removed before the patient is wrapped in thick blankets. Hot drinks do not help and should be avoided. Shivering is a good prognostic sign. Attempts to measure core temperature at the scene are pointless.

Post-immersion collapse

It requires at least two adults to lift a person from the water into a boat. Head-out upright immersion in water at body temperature results in a 32-66% increase in cardiac output because of the pressure of the surrounding water. On leaving the water this resistance to circulation is suddenly removed and, when added to venous pooling, the post-immersion circulatory collapse that occurs is believed to be the cause of death in many individuals found conscious in cold water but who perish within minutes of rescue. To counter this, it is recommended that patients be lifted out of the water in the prone position.

Associated injuries

Patients recovered from shallow water, particularly those with head injuries, often have an associated fracture or dislocation of the cervical spine. Those that have entered the water from a height may also suffer intra-abdominal and thoracic or spinal injuries (or both).

Resuscitation

Circulatory arrest should be managed in a unit in which facilities are available for bypass and extracorporeal rewarming. Therefore, a decision to intubate and selection of the target hospital is therefore taken on scene but practical difficulties mean that venous or arterial canulation is better left until arrival in hospital. Continuous chest compression should be applied without rewarming throughout transportation.

The role of procedures that are intended to drain water from the lungs and airways is controversial. Placing the patient's

> A fit young woman was cross-country skiing with friends, when she fell down a water-filled gully and became trapped beneath an ice sheet. Frantic efforts were made to extract her, but after 40 minutes, all movements ceased. Her body was eventually recovered, one hour and 19 minutes later, through a hole cut in the ice downstream. She was pronounced dead at the scene, but cardiopulmonary resuscitation was administered throughout the air-ambulance flight back to hospital, where her rectal temperature was recorded to be 13.7°C. Her body was rewarmed by means of an extracorporeal membrane oxygenator. Then, after 35 days on a ventilator and a further five months of rehabilitation, she was able to resume her regular duties—as a hospital doctor

Essential factors concerning the immersion incident

Length of time submerged	Favourable outcome associated with submersion for less than five minutes
Quality of immediate resuscitation	Favourable outcome if heart beat can be restored at once
Temperature of the water	Favourable outcome associated with immersion in ice-cold water (below 5°C), especially infants
Shallow water	Consider fracture or dislocation of cervical spine
A buoyancy aid being used by the casualty	Likely to be profoundly hypothermic. The patient may not have aspirated water. See post-immersion collapse
Nature of the water (fresh or salt)	Ventilation/perfusion mismatch from fresh water inhalation more difficult to correct. Risk of infection from river water high. Consider leptospirosis

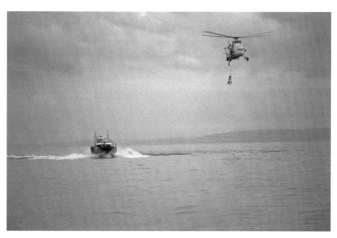

Rescue helicopter

head down in the lateral position probably only recovers water from the stomach. Aspiration of gastric contents is a constant hazard and is one of the reasons for attempting to intubate an unconscious patient at an early stage.

Hypothermia may render the carotid pulse impalpable, but it is important not to commence chest compression without evidence of cardiac arrest for fear of inducing ventricular fibrillation in a patient whose circulation, although sluggish, is otherwise intact. Electrocardiogram monitoring should be available. Defibrillation is ineffective if the myocardium is cold and there are obvious concerns for personal safety when discharging an electric charge in or around water. The bucking action of the craft makes expired air ventilation hazardous in an inshore rescue boat.

Management in hospital

Decision to admit
The decision to admit depends on whether water has been aspirated, because it is this that places the patient at risk from pulmonary oedema. Haemoptysis, lung crackles, fluffy shadows on the chest x ray, and hypoxia when breathing air are all signs of aspiration and are indications for hospital admission. If pulmonary oedema develops, it usually does so within four hours. Therefore, if after four hours the patient remains free of symptoms, he or she may be discharged home safely.

Pulmonary oedema and positive end expiratory pressure
A low reading thermometer with a rectal probe inserted at least 10 cm is often used to measure the patient's core temperature. Devices that measure the temperature of the tympanic membrane are a satisfactory alternative, provided that the patient's temperature is within the range of the device used. In the presence of a low core temperature a correction factor is required to calculate the true arterial blood oxygen saturation. A falling arterial PaO_2 level is a sign of impending respiratory distress syndrome ("normal atrial pressure pulmonary oedema") and an indication for assisted ventilation with positive end expiratory pressure (PEEP). The ideal pressure setting for PEEP is that which maintains the PaO_2 above 10 kPa, with an inspired oxygen fraction (FiO_2) below 0.6. Evidence suggests that aspirated fresh water is more likely than seawater to produce pulmonary oedema. Systemic steroids have no effect on outcome and offer no advantage.

Rewarming
Extracorporeal membrane oxygenation with extracorporeal warming is the gold standard treatment for patients with profound hypothermia. The Swiss Mountain Rescue Service has recovered the bodies of 46 individuals over the years, all with deep hypothermia from burial in snow. Fifteen out of 32 treated with extracorporeal rewarming survived. Conscious patients can be placed in a bath maintained at a temperature of 42°C.

Fluid and electrolyte balance
Plasma electrolyte differences between patients who aspire fresh water and seawater are seldom clinically important. In either situation, the patient is often hypovolaemic and in need of intravenous fluid replacement, preferably using a crystalloid. Metabolic acidosis should be corrected by adequate oxygenation and plasma expansion; administration of sodium bicarbonate should be unnecessary. Water intoxication resulting in fits has been reported in infants after near drowning in backyard pools.

Hypothermia
- Rewarm in bath water at 40°C
- Remove wet clothing if casualty can be sheltered
- Actively rewarm with extracorporeal bypass if necessary

Essential early measures

Tracheal intubation for unconscious patients	Secures the airway in the event of regurgitation
Electrocardiogram	Pulseless patient may have bradyarrhythmias or ventricular fibrillation
Nasogastric tube	Decompresses the stomach thereby assisting ventilation. Reduces the risk of regurgitation
Rectal temperature	Use low reading thermometer. Insert the probe at least 10 cm
Arterial blood gases	Low PaO_2 breathing air is a marker for pulmonary oedema or atelectasis with shunting. A pH less than 7 is associated with poor prognosis
Chest x ray examination	Shows aspirated fluid. Early indication of pulmonary oedema
Central venous line	Essential for monitoring level of positive end-expiratory pressure respiration
Culture blood for both aerobic and anaerobic organisms	Septicaemia common. Consider "exotic" organisms. Brain abscess is a late complication

---

Further measures
- Measure arterial gases: ensure low temperature correction
- In case of hypothermia raise core temperature above 28°C before defibrillation
- Consider plasma expanders and prophylactic antibiotics

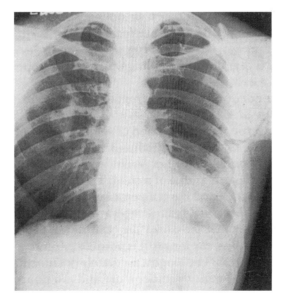

Shadowing in the left lower zone and right mid-zone represents aspirated water. The patient is at the risk of developing adult respiratory distress syndrome

Infection

Lung infection is common after near drowning, especially if brackish water has been aspirated. Embolism of infected material from the lungs to the arterial tree may result in brain abscesses or death from systemic aspergillosis. A blood culture should be undertaken in all instances in which aspiration has occurred. Leptospirosis has been reported after immersion in lakes or reservoirs, possibly due to ingestion of water contaminated with rats' urine. Outpatient follow-up with a chest x ray taken two weeks later is advisable for all patients who have been immersed in water, irrespective of their clinical state on admission.

Prognostic signs

A pH of 7 or less indicates severe acidosis and is a poor prognostic sign. A low PaO_2 provides an early indication that water has been inhaled with the attendant risk of pulmonary oedema. The presence of ventricular fibrillation is an adverse sign and responds poorly to defibrillation when the core temperature is below 28°C. The circulation must be supported by chest compression until further attempts can be made when the core temperature has been raised above this level.

Resuscitation on scene

- Chest compression alone for circulatory arrest
- No re-warming for deep hypothermia
- Intubate unconscious patients
- Defibrillation is unlikely to succeed
- Associated trauma may include fracture of the cervical spine

---

Resuscitation in hospital

- Aspiration is an indication for admission
- Facilities for extracorporeal blood re-warming should be available
- Correct arterial blood gas measurements for low core temperature
- Pulmonary oedema seldom develops later than four hours after immersion
- Blood-born sepsis is a late complication

Further reading

- Gilbert M, Busund R, Skagseth A, Nilsen PA, Solb. JP. Resuscitation from accidental hypothermia of 13.7°C with cardiac arrest. *Lancet* 2000;355:375-6.
- Golden FStC, Hervey GR, Tipton MJ. Circum-rescue collapse, sometimes fatal, associated with rescue of immersion victims. *J Roy Nav Med Serv* 1991;77:139.
- Golden FStC. Immersion in cold water: effects on performance and safety. In: Harries MJ, Williams C, Stanish WD Michaeli-Lyle J. eds. *Oxford textbook of sports medicine*, 2nd ed. Oxford: Oxford University Press, 1998:241-54.
- Orlowski JP, Abulleli MM, Phillips JM. Effects of tonicities of saline solutions on pulmonary injury in drowning. *Crit Care Med* 1987;1:126.
- Walpoth BH, Walpoth-Aslan BN, Mattle HP, Radanov BP, Schroth G, Schaeffler L, et al. Outcome of survivors of accidental deep hypothermia and circulatory arrest treated with extracorporeal blood warming. *N Engl J Med* 1997;337:500-5.

16 Drugs and their delivery

Michael Colquhoun, David Pitcher, Jerry Nolan

Drugs are given for several purposes during resuscitation attempts, but their use is largely empirical because it is thought that the known pharmacological actions of a drug might be beneficial. Much of the experimental evidence on the role of drugs has been derived from animal work, but the results have often been contradictory and the applicability of animal data to human cardiopulmonary resuscitation (CPR) is unclear. Controlled, prospective studies of the use of drugs in the clinical practice of resuscitation are difficult to perform and few have been carried out; in most cases such trials have raised doubts about the value of drugs rather than provided evidence of any benefit.

Current resuscitation guidelines recommend that drugs should be used when scientific evidence shows that drugs are of value, rather than for historical or theoretical reasons, or on the basis of anecdotal evidence alone. In many cases the strength of the evidence of benefit is inadequate to make a definite recommendation. In most cases, guidance represents a compromise between the available scientific evidence and a consensus view of experts who have reviewed that evidence.

This chapter is concerned with the principal drugs used during resuscitation attempts and in the peri-arrest situation when drug treatment, especially of cardiac rhythm disturbance, may prevent cardiac arrest. The routes by which drugs may be administered in these circumstances are also described.

Routes of Drug administration

Intravenous routes
Peripheral venous cannulation is safe, easily learned, and does not require interruption of CPR. It may, however, be difficult in hypovolaemic or obese patients. A large vein, usually in the antecubital fossa, is the site of choice, and drugs injected here during CPR reach peak concentration in the major systemic arteries 1.5-3 minutes later. This circulation time is reduced if the bolus of drug is followed by a normal saline flush, so once a cannula is in place it should be connected to an intravenous infusion that can be run in rapidly to aid drug administration. Raising the limb and massaging the veins will also speed delivery to the central circulation.

Central venous cannulation allows drugs to reach their site of action more rapidly and in a higher concentration, but the technique requires greater skill. It is particularly useful when cannulation of peripheral veins is technically difficult. The internal jugular and subclavian veins are most often used. The femoral vein is also available and this option is often forgotten. Subclavian cannulation requires interruption of chest compressions.

Endobronchial route
Tracheal intubation is performed at an early stage during some resuscitation attempts, and the endobronchial route may be the first available for the administration of drugs.

It is not the route of first choice and evidence of the efficiency of this method is conflicting. Endobronchial drugs

---

Complications of central venous cannulation

They include:
- Haemorrhage
- Arterial puncture
- Extravascular drug administration regardless of the vein used
- Pneumothorax if cannulation of the subclavian vein is attempted

Central venous cannulation may be hazardous after the administration of thrombolytic drugs, and, if required, in this circumstance the femoral approach is recommended. A wide-bore cannula placed in the antecubital fossa through which drugs may be flushed with normal saline seems to be the best route in clinical practice, at least during the early stages of most resuscitation attempts

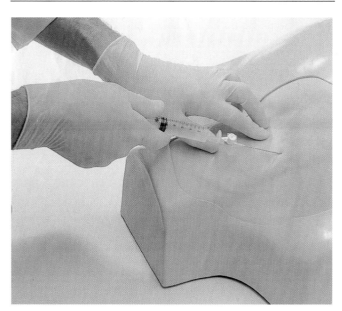

Central venous cannulation can be practised on a manikin

Adminstration of drugs via the endobronchial route
- Adrenaline (epinephrine), atropine, naloxone, and lidocaine (lignocaine) may be given by this route; the recommended doses are double those given intravenously
- The drugs should be diluted to a total volume of 10 ml with sterile water or isotonic saline and injected through a catheter passed beyond the tip of the tracheal tube; their rate of absorption will depend on the efficiency of CPR and will be reduced in the presence of pulmonary oedema

should only be given through a correctly sited tracheal tube and should not be given through other airway management devices, such as the laryngeal mask or Combi-tube.

Intraosseous route

Venous sinusoids in the intramedullary canal drain directly into the central circulation. Drugs may be given through a special intraosseous cannula inserted into the proximal tibia (2 cm below the tibial tuberosity on the anteromedial side) or distal tibia (2 cm proximal to the medial malleolus). This technique is used particularly in children, but it is also effective in adults.

> Any drug that can be given intravenously can also be given by the intraosseous route; the doses are the same as for the intravenous route

Anti-arrhythmic drugs

Two serious concerns about the use of anti-arrhythmic drugs are especially applicable to their use during resuscitation attempts and the period immediately after resuscitation. The first is their potential to provoke potentially dangerous cardiac arrhythmia as well as suppressing some abnormal rhythms—the "pro-arrhythmic" effect, which varies from drug to drug.

The second concern is the negative inotropic effect possessed by nearly all anti-arrhythmic drugs. This is of particular importance in the context of resuscitation attempts because myocardial function is often already compromised.

> Anti-arrhythmic drugs may be used in resuscitation attempts to terminate life-threatening cardiac arrhythmia, to facilitate electrical defibrillation, and to prevent recurrence of arrhythmia after successful defibrillation

Lidocaine (lignocaine)

Lidocaine is the anti-arrhythmic drug that has been studied most extensively. It has been used to treat ventricular tachycardia (VT) and ventricular fibrillation (VF) and to prevent recurrences of these arrhythmias after successful resuscitation. Several trials have shown that lidocaine is effective in preventing VF after acute myocardial infarction but no reduction in mortality has been shown, probably because the trials were conducted in a setting in which defibrillation was readily available to reverse VF if it occurred. It is no longer recommended for use in these circumstances.

Its role in the prevention of ventricular arrhythmia has been extended to the treatment of VF, particularly when used as an adjunct to electrical defibrillation—for example, when VF persists after initial DC shocks. Animal studies have shown that lidocaine increases the threshold for VF. However, the results may have been influenced by the experimental techniques used, and may not apply in humans. In one randomised, placebo-controlled trial a beneficial effect was seen on the defibrillation threshold, albeit in the special circumstance of patients undergoing coronary artery surgery. One clinical trial in humans showed a threefold greater occurrence of asystole after defibrillation when lidocaine had been given beforehand.

A recent systematic review concluded that the evidence supporting the efficacy of lidocaine was poor. The evidence supporting amiodarone was stronger and sufficient to recommend the use of amiodarone in preference to lidocaine in the treatment of shock-refractory VF and pulseless VT. On the basis of established use, lidocaine remains an acceptable, alternative treatment for VT and shock refractory VF/VT when adverse signs are absent. Current evidence, however, suggests that lidocaine is very much a drug of second choice behind amiodarone in these circumstances.

Amiodarone

Amiodarone is effective in the treatment of both supraventricular and ventricular arrhythmias. The main anti-arrhythmic action of amiodarone arises from its ability to prolong the duration of the myocardial action potential and

Administration of lidocaine
- It is given as a bolus (1.0-1.5 mg/kg) intravenously to achieve therapeutic levels
- A second dose of 0.5-0.75 mg/kg may be given over three to five minutes if the arrhythmia proves refractory, but the total dose should not exceed 3 mg/kg (or more than 200-300 mg) during the first hour of treatment
- If the arrhythmia responds to lidocaine it is common practice to try to maintain therapeutic levels using an infusion at 1-4 mg/min
- The difference between therapeutic and toxic plasma concentrations is small, so patients must be observed carefully for toxicity including slurred speech, depressed consciousness, muscular twitching, and fits

Administration of amiodarone
- In cardiac arrest amiodarone is given intravenously as a 300 mg bolus diluted in 20 ml of 5% dextrose or from a pre-filled syringe
- A further bolus of 150 mg may be given for recurrent or refractory VF and VT, followed by an infusion of 1 mg/min for six hours, followed by 0.5 mg/minute up to a maximum dose of 2 g in the first 24 hours

thereby increase cardiac refractoriness (Class 3). It is a complex drug with several other pharmacological effects, including minor α and β adrenoceptor blocking actions.

No strong evidence recommends the use of one particular anti-arrhythmic drug during cardiopulmonary arrest. However, on the basis of a single prospective, randomised, controlled trial (ARREST study), amiodarone was recommended as first choice for shock refractory VF and VT in the 2000 Resuscitation Guidelines. Since then, a prospective randomised trial (ALIVE trial) showed that, compared with lidocaine, treatment with amiodarone led to substantially higher rates of survival to hospital admission in patients with shock-resistant VF. The trial was not designed to have adequate statistical power to show an improvement in survival to hospital discharge. Amiodarone has the additional advantage of being the only currently available anti-arrhythmic drug to possess no substantial negative inotropic effect.

Flecainide
A potent sodium channel blocking drug (Class 1c) that results in substantial slowing of conduction of the action potential. It has proved effective in the termination of atrial flutter, atrial fibrillation (including pre-excited atrial fibrillation), VT, atrioventricular nodal re-entrant tachycardia (AVNRT), and junctional tachycardia associated with accessory pathway conduction (AVRT). Flecainide is currently included in the peri-arrest arrhythmia algorithm for atrial fibrillation. It is effective in the treatment of ventricular tachyarrhythmia but its place in resuscitation in this role is undetermined at present.

Bretylium
Bretylium has been used in the treatment of refractory VF and VT but no evidence shows its superiority over other drugs. Its anti-arrhythmic action is slow in onset and its other pharmacological effects, including adrenergic neurone blockade, result in hypotension that may be severe. Because of the high incidence of adverse effects, the availability of safer drugs that are at least as effective, and the limited availability of the drug, it has been removed from current resuscitation algorithms and guidelines.

β adrenoceptor blocking agents

These drugs (Class 2) are widely used in the treatment of patients with acute coronary syndromes and are given to the majority of such patients in the absence of contra-indications. β blocking drugs may reduce the incidence of VF in this situation and reduce mortality when given intravenously in the early stages of acute infarction. The main benefit is due to the prevention of ventricular rupture rather than the prevention of ventricular arrhythmias.

Esmolol
A short acting β1 receptor blocking drug currently included in the treatment algorithm for narrow complex tachycardia, which may be used to control the rate of ventricular response to atrial fibrillation or atrial flutter. It has a complicated dosing regimen and requires slow intravenous infusion.

Sotalol
A non-selective β blocker with additional Class 3 activity that prolongs the duration of the action potential and increases cardiac refractoriness. It may be given by slow intravenous infusion, but it is not readily available as an injectable preparation. Large doses are required to produce useful

Class 3 effects and are poorly tolerated because of fatigue or bradycardia due to its non-selective β blocking actions. Pro-arrhythmic actions may also occur, which may cause the torsades de pointes type of polymorphic VT.

Calcium channel blocking drugs

Verapamil and diltiazem are calcium channel blocking drugs that slow atrio-ventricular conduction by increasing refractoriness in the AV node. These actions may terminate or modify the behaviour of re-entry tachycardia involving the AV node, and may help to control the rate of ventricular response in patients with atrial fibrillation or flutter. Both drugs have strong negative inotropic actions that may precipitate or worsen cardiac failure, and both have largely been replaced in the treatment of regular narrow complex tachyarrhythmia by adenosine. Intravenous verapamil is contraindicated in patients taking β blockers because severe hypotension, bradycardia, or even asystole may result.

Adenosine

Adenosine is the drug of choice in the treatment of supraventricular tachycardia due to a re-entry pathway that includes the AV node. Adenosine produces transient AV block and usually terminates such arrhythmias. The half-life of the drug is very short (about 15 seconds) and its side effects of flushing, shortness of breath, and chest discomfort, although common, are short lived. If an arrhythmia is not due to a re-entry circuit involving the AV node—for example, atrial flutter or atrial fibrillation—it will not be terminated by adenosine but the drug may produce transient AV block that slows the rate of ventricular response and helps clarify the atrial rhythm. Adenosine should be given in an initial dose of 6 mg as a rapid intravenous bolus given as quickly as possible followed by a rapid saline flush. If no response is observed within one to two minutes a 12 mg dose is given in the same manner. Because of the short half-life of the drug the arrhythmia may recur and repeat episodes may be treated with additional doses, intravenous esmolol, or with verapamil. An intravenous infusion of amiodarone is an alternative strategy.

Atropine

Atropine antagonises the parasympathetic neurotransmitter acetylcholine at muscarinic receptors; its most clinically important effects are on the vagus nerve. By decreasing vagal tone on the heart, sinus node automaticity is increased and AV conduction is facilitated. Increased parasympathetic tone—for example, after acute inferior myocardial infarction—may lead to bradyarrhythmias such as sinus bradycardia, AV block, or asystole; atropine is often an effective treatment in this setting.

Atropine may sometimes be beneficial in the treatment of AV block. This is particularly so in the presence of a narrow complex escape rhythm arising high in the conducting system. Complete heart block with a slow broad complex idioventricular escape rhythm is much less likely to respond to atropine. The recommended treatment is an initial dose of 500 mcg intravenously, repeated after 3-5 minutes as necessary up to a maximum dose of 3.0 mg.

Atropine is most effective in the treatment of asystolic cardiac arrest when this is due to profound vagal discharge. It has been widely used to treat asystole when the cause is uncertain, but it has never been proved to be of value in this situation; such evidence that exists is limited to small series and case reports. Asystole carries a grave prognosis, however, and anecdotal accounts of successful resuscitation after atropine, and its lack of adverse effects, lead to its continued use. In asystole it should be given only once as a dose of 3 mg intravenously, which will produce full vagal blockade.

Magnesium

Magnesium deficiency, like hypokalaemia with which it often coexists, may be caused by long-term diuretic treatment, pre-dispose a patient to ventricular arrhythmias and sudden cardiac death, and cause refractory VF.

Catecholamines and Vasopressin

Catecholamines

Coronary blood flow during closed chest CPR is determined by the pressure gradient across the myocardial circulation, which is the difference between aortic and right atrial pressure. By producing vasoconstriction in the peripheral circulation catecholamines and other vasopressor drugs raise the aortic pressure, thereby increasing coronary and cerebral perfusion. Much evidence from experimental work in animals shows that these actions increase the likelihood of successful resuscitation. In spite of this, adrenaline (epinephrine) does not improve survival or neurological recovery in humans. Adrenaline (epinephrine) is the drug currently recommended in the management of all forms of cardiac arrest.

Pending definitive placebo-controlled trials, the indications, dose, and time interval between doses of adrenaline (epinephrine) have not changed. In practical terms, for non-VF/VT rhythms each "loop" of the algorithm (see Chapter 3) lasts three minutes and, therefore, adrenaline (epinephrine) is given with every loop. For shockable rhythms the process of rhythm assessment and the administration of three shocks followed by one minute of CPR will take between two and three minutes. Therefore, adrenaline (epinephrine) should be given with each loop.

Experimental work in animals has suggested potential advantages from larger doses of adrenaline (epinephrine) than those currently used. Small case series and retrospective studies of higher doses after human cardiac arrest have reported favourable outcomes. Clinical trials conducted in the early 1990s showed that the use of higher doses (usually 5 mg) of adrenaline (epinephrine) (compared with the standard dose of 1 mg) was associated with a higher rate of return of spontaneous circulation. However, no substantial improvement in the rate of survival to hospital discharge was seen, and high-dose adrenaline (epinephrine) is not recommended.

Adrenaline (epinephrine) may also be used in patients with symptomatic bradycardia if both atropine and transcutaneous pacing (if available) fail to produce an adequate increase in heart rate.

Vasopressin

Preliminary clinical studies suggest that vasopressin may increase the chance of restoring spontaneous circulation in humans with out-of-hospital VF. Animal studies, and the clinical evidence that exists, suggest that it may be particularly useful when the duration of cardiac arrest is prolonged. In these circumstances the vasoconstrictor response to adrenaline (epinephrine) is attenuated in the presence of substantial acidosis, whereas the response to vasopressin is unchanged.

Magnesium treatment

- Magnesium deficiency should be corrected if known to be present
- 2 g of magnesium sulphate is best given as an infusion over 10-20 minutes, but in an emergency it may be given as an undiluted bolus
- Magnesium is an effective treatment for drug-induced torsades de pointes, even in the absence of demonstrable magnesium deficiency
- One suitable regimen is an initial dose of 1-2 g (8-16 mEq) diluted in 50-100 ml of 5% dextrose administered over 5-60 minutes
- Thereafter, an infusion of 0.5-1.0 g/hour is given; the rate and duration of the infusion is determined by the clinical situation

---

Potassium

Hypokalaemia, like magnesium deficiency, pre-disposes cardiac arrhythmia. Diuretic therapy is the commonest cause of potassium depletion. This may be exacerbated by the action of endogenous or administered catecholamines, which stimulate potassium uptake into cells at the expense of extracellular potassium. Hypokalaemia is more common in patients taking regular diuretic therapy and is associated with a higher incidence of VF after myocardial infarction; correction of hypokalaemia reduces the risk of cardiac arrest. When VT or VF is resistant to defibrillation, despite the use of amiodarone, the possibility of severe hypokalaemia is worth investigating and treating

---

Actions of catecholamines

- Within the vascular smooth muscle of the peripheral resistance vessels, both $\alpha 1$ and $\alpha 2$ receptors produce vasoconstriction
- During hypoxic states it is thought that the $\alpha 1$ receptors become less potent and that $\alpha 2$ adrenergic receptors contribute more towards maintaining vasomotor tone. This may explain the ineffectiveness of pure $\alpha 1$ agonists, whereas adrenaline (epinephrine) and noradrenaline (norepinephrine), which both possess $\alpha 1$ and $\alpha 2$ agonist action, have been shown to enhance coronary perfusion pressure considerably during cardiac arrest
- The $\alpha 2$ agonist activity seems to become increasingly important as the duration of circulatory arrest progresses
- The β agonist activity (which both drugs possess) seems to have a beneficial effect, at least partly by counteracting $\alpha 2$-mediated coronary vasoconstriction
- Several clinical trials have compared different catecholamine-like drugs in the treatment of cardiac arrest but none has been shown to be more effective than adrenaline (epinephrine), which, therefore, remains the drug of choice

---

Actions of adrenaline (epinephrine)

- Stimulates $\alpha 1$, $\alpha 2$, $\beta 1$, and $\beta 2$ receptors
- The vasoconstrictor effect on α receptors is thought to be beneficial
- The β stimulation may be detrimental
- Increased heart rate and force of contraction results, thereby raising myocardial oxygen requirements
- Increased glycogenolysis increases oxygen requirements and produces hypokalaemia, with an increased chance of arrhythmia
- To avoid the potentially detrimental β effects, selective $\alpha 1$ agonists have been investigated but have been found to be ineffective in clinical use

In one small study of 40 patients, more patients treated with vasopressin were successfully resuscitated and survived for 24 hours compared with those who received adrenaline (epinephrine); no difference in survival to hospital discharge was noted. In another study, 200 patients with in-hospital cardiac arrest (all rhythms) were given either vasopressin 40 U or adrenaline (epinephrine) 1 mg as the initial vasopressor. Forty members (39%) of the vasopressin group survived for one hour compared with 34 (35%) members of the adrenaline (epinephrine) group (P = 0.66). A European multicentre out-of-hospital study to determine the effect of vasopressin versus adrenaline (epinephrine) on short-term survival has almost finished recruiting the planned 1500 patients.

The International Resuscitation Guidelines 2000 recommend using vasopressin as an alternative to adrenaline (epinephrine) for the treatment of shock-refractory VF in adults. Not all experts agree with this decision and the Advanced Life Support Working Group of the European Resuscitation Council (ERC) has not included vasopressin in the ERC Guidelines 2000 for adult advanced life support.

Inadequate data support the use of vasopressin in patients with asystole or pulseless electrical activity (PEA) or in infants and children.

Calcium

Calcium has a vital role in cardiac excitation–contraction coupling mechanisms. However, a considerable amount of evidence suggests that its use during cardiac arrest is ineffective and possibly harmful.

Neither serum nor tissue calcium concentrations fall after cardiac arrest; bolus injections of a calcium salts increase intracellular calcium concentrations and may produce myocardial necrosis or uncontrolled myocardial contraction. Smooth muscle in peripheral arteries may also contract in the presence of high calcium concentrations and further reduce blood flow. The brain is particularly susceptible to this action.

Alkalising drugs

The return of spontaneous circulation and adequate ventilation is the best way to ensure correction of the acid-base disturbances that accompany cardiopulmonary arrest.

During cardiac arrest gas exchange in the lungs ceases, whereas cellular metabolism continues in an anaerobic environment; this produces a combination of respiratory and metabolic acidosis. The most effective treatment for this condition (until spontaneous circulation can be restored) is chest compression to maintain the circulation and ventilation to provide oxygen and remove carbon dioxide.

Sodium bicarbonate

Much of the evidence about the use of sodium bicarbonate has come from animal work, and both positive and negative results have been reported; the applicability of these results to humans is questionable. No adequate prospective studies have been performed to investigate the effect of sodium bicarbonate on the outcome of cardiac arrest in humans, and retrospective studies have focused on patients with prolonged arrests in whom resuscitation was unlikely to be successful. Advantages have been reported in relation to a reduction in defibrillation thresholds, higher rates of return of spontaneous circulation, a reduced incidence of recurrent VF, and an increased rate of hospital discharge. Benefit seems most probable when the dose

---

Action of vasopressin (the natural anti-diuretic hormone)

- In pharmacological doses, it acts as a potent peripheral vasoconstrictor, producing effects by direct stimulation of V1 receptors on smooth muscle
- The half-life of vasopressin is about 20 minutes, which is considerably longer than that of adrenaline (epinephrine). In experimental animals in VF or with PEA vasopressin increased coronary perfusion pressure, blood flow to vital organs, and cerebral oxygen delivery
- Unlike adrenaline (epinephrine), vasopressin does not increase myocardial oxygen consumption during CPR because it is devoid of β agonist activity
- After administration of vasopressin the receptors on vascular smooth muscle produce intense vasoconstriction in the skin, skeletal muscle, and intestine
- Release of endothelial nitric oxide prevents vasopressin-induced constriction of coronary, cerebral, and renal vessels

---

On the basis of the evidence from animal work and clinical studies the use of calcium is not recommended in the treatment of asystole or PEA, except in known cases of hypocalcaemia or hyperkalaemia or when calcium channel blockers have been administered in excessive doses

---

Sodium bicarbonate in cardiac arrest

- Bicarbonate exacerbates intracellular acidosis because the carbon dioxide that it generates diffuses rapidly into cells; the effects may be particularly marked in the brain, which lacks the phosphate and protein buffers found in other tissues
- The accumulation of carbon dioxide in the myocardium causes further depression of myocardial contractility
- An increase in pH will shift the oxygen dissociation curve to the left, further inhibiting release of oxygen from haemoglobin
- Sodium bicarbonate solution is hyperosmolar in the concentrations usually used and the sodium load may exacerbate cerebral oedema
- In the experimental setting hyperosmolarity is correlated with reduced aortic pressure and a consequential reduction in coronary perfusion

---

Alternatives to sodium bicarbonate

- These include tris hydroxymethyl aminomethane (THAM), Carbicarb (equimolar combination of sodium bicarbonate and sodium carbonate), and tribonate (a combination of THAM, sodium acetate, sodium bicarbonate, and sodium phosphate)
- Each has the advantage of producing little or no carbon dioxide, but studies have not shown consistent benefits over sodium bicarbonate

of bicarbonate is titrated to replenish the bicarbonate ion and given concurrently with adrenaline (epinephrine), the effect of which is enhanced by correction of the pH.

In the past, infusion of sodium bicarbonate has been advocated early in cardiac arrest in an attempt to prevent or reverse acidosis. Its action as a buffer depends on the excretion of the carbon dioxide generated from the lungs, but this is limited during cardiopulmonary arrest. Only judicious use of sodium bicarbonate can be recommended, and correction of acidosis should be based on determinations of pH and base excess. Arterial blood is not suitable for these measurements; central venous blood samples better reflect tissue acidosis.

It has been recommended that sodium bicarbonate should be considered at a pH of less than 7.0-7.1 ([H]-1 > 80 mmol/l) with a base excess of less than −10; however, the general level of acidosis is not generally agreed upon. Doses of 50 mmol of bicarbonate should be titrated against the pH. On the basis of the potentially detrimental effects described above, many clinicians rarely give bicarbonate. However, it is indicated for cardiac arrest associated with hyperkalaemia or with tricyclic antidepressant overdose.

Pharmacological approaches to cerebral protection after cardiac arrest

The cerebral ischaemia that follows cardiac arrest results in the rapid exhaustion of cerebral oxygen, glucose, and high-energy phosphates. Cell membranes start to leak almost immediately and cerebral oedema results. Calcium channels in the cell membranes open, calcium flows into the cells, and this triggers a cascade of events that result in neuronal damage. If resuscitation is successful, reperfusion of the cerebral circulation can damage nerve cells further. Several mechanisms for this have been proposed, including vasospasm, red cell sludging, hypermetabolic states, and acidosis.

Treatment of cerebral oedema
Immediately after the return of spontaneous circulation cerebral hyperaemia occurs. After 15-30 minutes of reperfusion global cerebral blood flow decreases, which is due, in part to cerebral oedema, with resulting cerebral hypoperfusion. Pharmacological measures to reduce cerebral oedema, including the use of diuretics, may exacerbate the period of hypoperfusion and should be avoided. Corticosteroids increase the risk of infection and gastric haemorrhage, and raise blood glucose concentration but no evidence has been found to support their use.

Calcium channel blockers
Because of the role that calcium may play in causing neuronal injury, calcium channel blocking drugs have been investigated for their possible protective effect both in animal experiments and in several clinical trials. No drug, including lidoflazine, nimodipine, flunarizine, or nicardipine, has been found to be beneficial. Several different calcium entry channels exist and only the voltage-dependent L type is blocked by the drugs studied, so excess calcium entry may not have been prevented under the trial conditions.

Excitatory amino acid receptor antagonists
Recently, the excitatory amino acid neurotransmitters (especially glutamate and aspartate) have been implicated in causing neuronal necrosis after ischaemia. The N-methyl-D-aspartate (NMDA) receptor, which has a role in controlling calcium influx into the cell, has been studied, but unfortunately no benefit from specific NMDA receptor antagonists has been seen.

Free radicals
Oxygen-derived free radicals have been implicated in the production of ischaemic neuronal damage. During both ischaemia and reperfusion the natural free radical scavengers are depleted. In certain experimental settings exogenous free radical scavengers (desferrioxamine, superoxide dismutase, and catalase) have been shown to influence an ischaemic insult to the brain, suggesting a potential use for these drugs, although no clear role in clinical practice has currently been defined.

> Early attempts at cerebral protection aimed at reproducing the depression in brain metabolism seen in hypothermia, and barbiturate anaesthesia was investigated for this purpose. Two recent studies have shown improved neurological outcome with the induction of mild hypothermia (33 °C) for 24 hours after cardiac arrest (see Chapter 7)

Summary
- The use of drugs in resuscitation attempts has only rarely been based on sound scientific or clinical trial evidence
- In most cases the rationale for their use has been based on animal work or anecdotes, or has developed empirically
- All drugs have a risk of adverse effects but the magnitude of these is often difficult to quantify
- Formal clinical evaluation in large prospective studies is required for all drugs, even those already in current use. The obstacles to such research are formidable but must be tackled so that future resuscitation practice can be based on sound scientific evidence
- Finally, remember that most patients who survive cardiac arrest are those who are defibrillated promptly; at best, pharmacological treatment retards the effects of hypoxia and acidosis until the cardiac rhythm can be restored.

Further reading
- Dorian P, Cass D, Schwartz B, Cooper R, Gelaznikas R, Barr A., et al. Amiodarone as compared with lidocaine for shock resistant ventricular fibrillation (ALIVE). *N Engl J Med* 2002;346:884-90.
- International guidelines 2000 for cardiopulmonary resuscitation and emergency cardiovascular care—an international consensus on science. Part 6 advanced cardiovascular life support. Section 5 pharmacology 1: agents for arrhythmias. *Resuscitation* 2000;46:135-53. Section 6 Pharmacology 2: Agents to optimize cardiac output and blood pressure. *Resuscitation* 2000;46:155-62.
- Kudenchuk PJ, Cobb LA, Copass MK, Cummins RO, Doherty AM, Farenbruch CE, et al. Amiodarone for resuscitation after out-of-hospital cardiac arrest due to ventricular fibrillation (ARREST). *N Engl J Med* 1999;341:871-8.

17 Cardiac pacing and implantable cardioverter defibrillators

Michael Colquhoun, A John Camm

Cardiac pacing

An artificial cardiac pacemaker is an electronic device that is designed to deliver a small electrical charge to the myocardium and thereby produce depolarisation and contraction of cardiac muscle. The charge is usually applied directly to the endocardium through transvenous electrodes; sometimes epicardial or oesophageal electrodes are used. They are all specialised invasive techniques and require considerable expertise and specialised equipment.

Non-invasive external pacing utilises cutaneous electrodes attached to the skin surface and provides a quick method of achieving pacing in an emergency situation. It is relatively easy to perform and can, therefore, be instigated by a wide range of personnel and used in environments in which invasive methods cannot be employed. Increasingly, the defibrillators used in the ambulance service and the coronary care unit incorporate the facility to use this type of pacing.

Pacemakers may be inserted as an interim measure to treat a temporary or self-limiting cardiac rhythm disturbance or implanted permanently when long-term treatment is required. A temporary pacing system is often inserted as a holding measure until definitive treatment is possible.

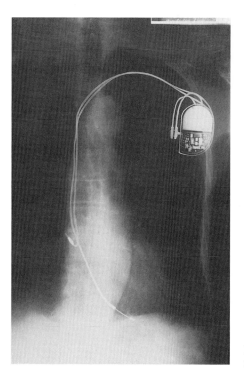

Dual chamber pacemaker in situ

Electrocardiogram appearances

The discharge from the pulse generator is usually a square wave that rises almost instantaneously to a preset output voltage, decays over the course of about 0.5 msec, then falls abruptly to zero. The conventional electrocardiogram (ECG) monitor or recorder cannot follow these rapid fluctuations and when the pacing stimulus is recorded it is usually represented as a single spike on the display or printout; some digital monitors may fail to record the spike at all. Although this spike may lack detail, recognition of a stimulus artefact is usually adequate for analysis of the cardiac rhythm.

Pacing modes

Two basic pacing modes are used. With fixed rate, or asynchronous, pacing the generator produces stimuli at regular intervals, regardless of the underlying cardiac rhythm. Unfortunately, competition between paced beats and the intrinsic cardiac rhythm may lead to irregular palpitation, and stimulation during ventricular repolarisation can lead to serious ventricular arrhythmias, including ventricular fibrillation (VF). This is not the pacing mode of choice.

With demand, or synchronous, pacing the generator senses spontaneous QRS complexes that inhibit its output. If the intrinsic cardiac rate is higher than the selected pacing rate then the generator will be inhibited completely. If a spontaneous QRS complex is not followed by another within a predetermined escape interval an impulse is generated. This mode of pacing minimises competition between natural and paced beats and reduces the risk of inducing arrhythmias.

Some pacemakers have an escape interval after a sensed event (the hysteresis interval) that is substantially longer than

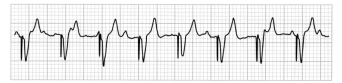

Ventricular pacing spikes seen before the QRS complex

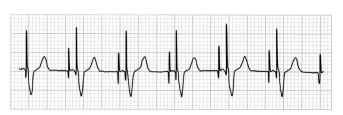

Atrial and ventricular pacing artefacts seen with dual chamber pacing

the automatic interval (the interval between two consecutive stimuli during continuous pacing). This may permit more spontaneous cardiac activity before the pacemaker fires. With temporary pacing systems a control on the pulse generator allows selection of the pacing mode; with permanent systems the unit may be converted from demand to fixed rate mode by placing a magnet over the generator.

Indications for pacing

The principal indication for pacing is bradycardia. This may arise because of failure of the sinoatrial node to generate an impulse or because failure of impulse conduction occurs in the atrioventricular (AV) node or His–Purkinje system. A permanent pacing system is most often used to treat sinus bradycardia, sinus arrest, and AV block.

Pacing is also used for tachycardia; a paced beat or sequence of beats is used to interrupt the tachycardia and provides an opportunity for sinus rhythm to become re-established. Atrial flutter and certain forms of junctional tachycardia may be terminated by atrial pacing. Ventricular burst pacing is sometimes used to treat ventricular tachycardia (VT), but this requires an implanted defibrillator to be used as a backup. Certain types of malignant ventricular arrhythmia may be prevented by accelerating the underlying heart rate by pacing; this is particularly valuable for preventing polymorphic VT.

Pacing during resuscitation attempts

In the context of resuscitation, pacing is most commonly used to treat bradycardia preceeding cardiac arrest or complications in the post-resuscitation period; complete (third-degree) AV block is the most important bradycardia in this situation.

Pacing may also be used as a preventive strategy when the occurrence of serious bradycardia or asystole can be anticipated. This is considered further in the section on the management of bradycardia (Chapter 5). One particularly important use is in patients with acute myocardial infarction (MI) in whom lesser degrees of conduction disturbance may precede the development of complete AV block; prophylactic temporary pacing should be considered in these circumstances.

Pacing is indicated in the treatment of asystolic cardiac arrest provided that some electrical activity, which may represent sporadic atrial or QRS complexes, is present. It is ineffective after VF has degenerated into terminal asystole.

Emergency cardiac pacing

Pacing must be instituted very quickly in the treatment or prevention of cardiac arrest. Although transvenous pacing is the ideal, it is seldom possible in the cardiac arrest setting, particularly outside hospital; even in hospital it takes time to arrange. Non-invasive pacing is quick and easy to perform and requires minimal training. Therefore, it is suitable to be used by a wide range of personnel including nurses and paramedics. Unfortunately, non-invasive pacing is not entirely reliable and is best considered to be a holding measure to allow time for the institution of temporary transvenous pacing.

External cardiac percussion is performed by administering firm blows at a rate of 100 per minute over the heart to the left of the lower sternum, although the exact spot in an individual patient usually has to be found by trial and error. The hand should fall a few inches only; the force used is less than a precordial thump and is usually tolerated by a conscious patient; it should be reduced to the minimum force required to produce a QRS complex.

Non-invasive methods

Fist or thump pacing

When pacing is indicated but cannot be instituted without a delay, external cardiac percussion (known as fist or thump

Principal indications for pacing

1. Third-degree (complete) AV block:
   - When pauses of three seconds or more or any escape rate of more than 40 beats/min or symptoms due to the block occur
   - Arrhythmias or other medical conditions requiring drugs that result in symptomatic bradycardia
   - After catheter ablation of the AV junction
   - Post-operative or post-MI AV block not expected to resolve
2. Sinus node dysfunction with:
   - Symptomatic bradycardia or pauses that produce symptoms
   - Chronotropic incompetence
3. Chronic bifascicular and trifascicular block associated with:
   - Intermittent third-degree AV block
   - Mobitz type II second-degree AV block
4. Hypersensitive carotid sinus syndrome and neurally mediated syncope
5. Tachycardias:
   - Symptomatic recurrent supraventricular tachycardia reproducibly terminated by pacing, after drugs and catheter ablation fail to control the arrhythmia or produce intolerable side effects
   - Sustained pause-dependent VT when pacing has been shown to be effective in prevention

Pacing may be used in the following conditions:

- Bradycardia preceding cardiac arrest
- Preventative strategy for serious bradycardia or asystole
- Acute MI
- Asystolic cardiac arrest

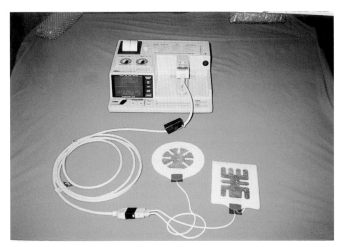

External cardiac pacemaker

pacing) may generate QRS complexes with an effective cardiac output, particularly when myocardial contractility is not critically compromised. Conventional cardiopulmonary resuscitation (CPR) should be substituted immediately if QRS complexes with a discernible output are not being achieved.

Transcutaneous external pacing

Many defibrillators incorporate external pacing units and use the same electrode pads for ECG monitoring and defibrillation. Alternatively, pacing may be the sole function of a dedicated external pacing unit. The pacing electrodes are attached to the patient's chest wall after suitable preparation of the skin, if time allows. The cathode should be in a position corresponding to V3 of the ECG and the anode on the left posterior chest wall beneath the scapula at the same level as the anterior electrode. This configuration is also appropriate for defibrillation and will not interfere with the subsequent placement of defibrillator electrodes in the conventional anterolateral position, should this be necessary.

Both defibrillation and pacing may be performed with electrodes placed in an anterolateral position, but the electrode position should be changed if a high pacing threshold or loss of capture occurs. It is important to ensure that the correct electrode polarity is employed, otherwise an unacceptably high pacing threshold may result. Modern units with integral cables that connect the electrodes to the pulse generator ensure the correct polarity, provided the electrodes are positioned correctly.

With the unit switched on, the pacing rate is selected (usually 60-90 per minute) and the demand mode is normally chosen if the machine has that capability. If electrical interference is substantial (as may arise from motion artefact), problems with sensing may occur and the unit may be inappropriately inhibited; in this case it is better to select the fixed rate mode. The fixed rate mode may also be required if the patient has a failing permanent pacemaker because the temporary system may be inhibited by the output from the permanent generator.

The pacing current is gradually increased from the minimum setting while carefully observing the patient and the ECG. A pacing artefact will be seen on the ECG monitor and, when capture occurs, it will be followed by a QRS complex, which is, in turn, followed by a T wave. Contraction of skeletal muscle on the chest wall may also be seen. The minimum current that achieves electrical capture is known as the pacing threshold, and a value above this is selected when the patient is paced. The presence of a palpable pulse confirms capture and mechanical contraction. Failure to achieve an output despite good electrical capture on the ECG is analogous to electromechanical dissociation, and an urgent search for correctable causes should be made before concluding that the myocardium is not viable.

When the external pacing unit is not part of a defibrillator, defibrillation may be performed in the conventional manner, but the defibrillator paddles should be placed as far as possible from the pacing electrodes to prevent electrical arcing.

Invasive methods

Temporary transvenous pacing

A bipolar catheter that incorporates two pacing electrodes at the distal end is introduced into the venous circulation and passed into the right ventricle. Pacing is performed once a stable position with an acceptable threshold has been found, usually at a site near the right ventricular apex. X ray screening is usually used to guide the placement of the pacing wire, but when this is not easily available flotation electrode systems, such

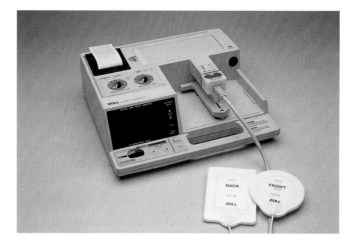

External pacemaker with electrodes

Pacing procedure

- Switch on unit
- Select pacing rate
- Choose demand mode if available
- Select fixed rate mode if significant interference, or if a failing permanent pacemaker
- Increase pacing current gradually observing patient and ECG
- Pacing artefact appears on ECG when capture occurs
- Minimum current to achieve capture is the pacing threshold

External pacing can be extremely uncomfortable for a conscious patient and sedation and analgesia may be required. Once successful pacing has been achieved, plans for the insertion of a transvenous system should be made without delay because external pacing is only a temporary measure

Chest compression can be performed with transcutaneous pacing electrodes in place. The person performing the compression is not at risk because the current energies are very small and the electrodes are well insulated. It is usual practice, however, to turn the unit off should CPR be required

as the Swan-Ganz catheter, that feature an inflatable balloon near the tip offer an alternative method of entering the right ventricle. A central vein, either the subclavian or jugular, is cannulated to provide access to the venous circulation. Manipulation of the catheter is easier than when peripheral venous access is used, and the risks of subsequent displacement are less. Full aseptic precautions must be used because the pacemaker may be required for several days and infection of the system may be disastrous.

Once a potentially suitable position has been found the pacing catheter/electrode is connected to a pulse generator and the pacing threshold (the minimum voltage that will capture the ventricle) is measured. This should be less than 1 volt, and the patient is paced at three times the threshold or 3 volts, whichever is the higher. If the threshold is high, the wire should be repositioned and the threshold measured again. Regular checks should be undertaken—a rise in threshold will indicate the development of exit block (failure of the pacing stimulus to penetrate the myocardium) or displacement of the pacing wire.

Defibrillation may be performed in patients fitted with a temporary transvenous pacing system but it is important that the defibrillator paddles do not come into contact with the temporary pacing wire and associated leads, and that electrical arcing to the pacing wire through conductive gel does not occur.

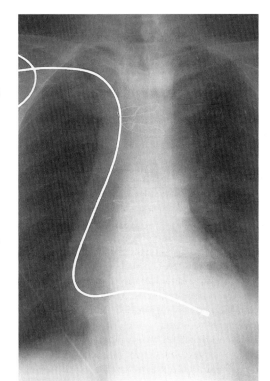

Temporary pacing wire in right ventricle

Permanent pacemakers

Modern permanent pulse generators are extremely sophisticated devices. Most use two leads to enable both sensing and pacing of the right atrium as well as the right ventricle. This allows both atrial and ventricular single-chamber pacing and dual-chamber pacing, in which both pacing and sensing can take place in the atrium and ventricle to allow more physiological cardiac stimulation.

Some devices also increase the rate of pacing automatically to match physiological demand. Modern generators are programmable, whereby an electromagnetic signal from an external programming device is used to modify one or more of the pacing functions. The optimal mode for the individual patient may be selected or the feature may be used to diagnose and treat certain pacing complications. External programming allows modifications of pacing characteristics or the incorporation of features that had not been anticipated at the time of implantation.

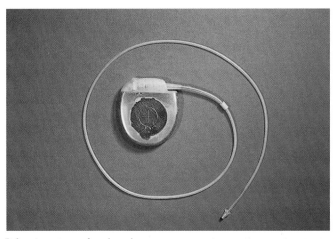

Pulse generator and pacing wire

Defibrillation and permanent pacemakers

The sophisticated electronics contained in modern pulse generators may be damaged by the output from a defibrillator, although a protection circuit contained in the generator helps to reduce this risk. Defibrillator electrodes should be placed as far as possible from a pacemaker generator, but at least 12.5 cm. To achieve this, it is often best to use the anteroposterior position.

If the generator has been put in the usual position below the left clavicle, the conventional anterolateral position may be suitable. After successful resuscitation the device should be checked to ensure that the programming has not been affected.

A further complication is that current from the defibrillator may travel down the pacing electrode and produce burns at the point at which the electrode tip lies against the myocardium.

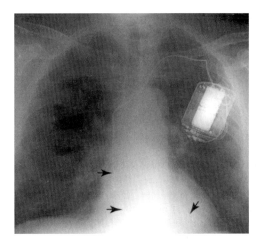

Chest radiograph showing biventricular pacemaker with leads in the right ventricle, right atrium, and coronary sinus (arrows)

This may result in a rise in the electrical threshold and loss of pacing. This complication may not become apparent until some time after the shock has been given. For this reason the pacing threshold should be checked regularly for several weeks after successful resuscitation.

The implantable cardioverter defibrillator

The implantable cardioverter defibrillator (ICD) was developed for the prevention of sudden cardiac death in patients with life-threatening ventricular arrhythmias, particularly sustained VT or VF. Observational studies and recent prospective studies have shown their effectiveness.

Technological advances have been rapid and modern cardioverter-defibrillators are much smaller than their predecessors. One or more electrodes are usually inserted transvenously, although a subcutaneous electrode is sometimes used. Some new designs use subcutaneous electrodes exclusively and are implanted over the heart; no transvenous or intracardiac electrodes are required.

Currently available models feature several tachycardia zones with rate detection criteria and tiered therapy (low-energy cardioversion and high-energy defibrillation shocks) independently programmable for each zone. All feature programmable ventricular demand pacing. Extensive diagnostic features are available, including stored ECGs of the rhythm before and after tachycardia detection and treatment. Programmable anti-tachycardia pacing is an option with many models.

Defibrillation is achieved by an electric charge applied between the anodal and cathodal electrodes. The site and number of anodes and cathodes, the shape of the shock waveform, and the timing and sequence of shocks can all be pre-programmed. Biphasic shocks (in which the polarity of the shock waveform reverses during the discharge) are widely used. The capacitors are charged from an integral battery, which takes 5-30 seconds after the recognition of the arrhythmia.

Implantable defibrillators incorporating an atrial lead are also available. These provide dual-chamber pacing and can also distinguish atrial from ventricular tachyarrhythmias. They are used in patients who require an ICD and concomitant dual-chamber pacing, and in patients with supraventricular tachycardias that may lead to inappropriate ICD discharge. Atrial defibrillators have also become available in recent years to treat paroxysmal atrial fibrillation. Detailed supervision and follow up are required with all devices.

Resuscitation in patients with an ICD

Should resuscitation be required in a patient with an ICD, basic life support should be carried out in the usual way. If defibrillation is attempted no substantial shock will be felt by the rescuer. If it is deemed necessary to turn the device off this may be accomplished by placing a magnet over the ICD. If external defibrillation is attempted the same precautions should be observed as for patients with pacemakers, placing the defibrillator electrodes as far from the unit as possible. If resuscitation is successful the ICD should be completely re-assessed to ensure that it has not been adversely affected by the shock from the external defibrillator.

Indications for implantation of an ICD

It is important to recognise those patients who are successfully resuscitated from cardiac arrest yet remain at risk of developing a further lethal arrhythmia. ICDs have been shown to be

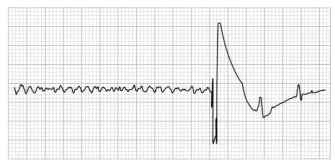

Defibrillation by an ICD

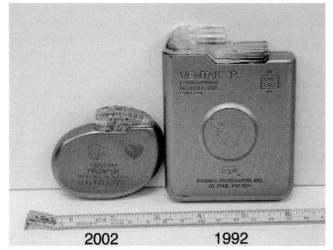

2002   1992

Changes in ICDs over 10 years (1992–2002). Apart from reduction in size, the implant technique and required hardware have also improved—from the sternotomy approach with four leads and abdominal implantation to the present two-lead transvenous endocardial approach that is no more invasive than a pacemaker requires

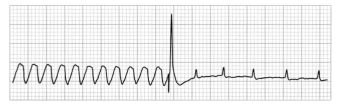

Cardioversion of ventricular tachycardia by an ICD

Abdominal insertion or thoracotomy (needed with earlier models) is rarely required because most devices are now placed in an infraclavicular position similar to that used for a pacemaker

ICDs for secondary prevention

- Cardiac arrest due to VT or VF
- Spontaneous VT causing syncope or significant haemodynamic compromise
- Sustained VT without syncope or cardiac arrest with an ejection rate of 35% but no worse than Classs 3 of the New York Heart Association classification of heart failure
- For patients who have not suffered life threatening arrhythmia but are at high risk of sudden cardiac death

effective in the prevention of sudden cardiac death in these patients and are, therefore, indicated as a "secondary" preventative measure. In clinical trials ICDs have been shown to be more effective than anti-arrhythmic drugs in this role.

All patients who are resuscitated from cardiac arrest due to VF or VT should routinely be considered for implantation of an ICD unless a treatable cause for the arrest is found. Similarly, ICDs should be routinely considered in patients with sustained VT leading to syncope or other substantial haemodynamic compromise, again unless a treatable cause is discovered.

Patients with severe impairment of left ventricular function have a high incidence of sudden cardiac death. Implantation of an ICD may be indicated as a preventative measure if the left ventricular ejection fraction is less than 35% and they have experienced an episode of sustained VT, even without syncope or cardiac arrest.

Patients resuscitated from VF occurring in the early stages of MI do not usually remain at risk of further episodes in the absence of other complications.

It is also possible to identify patients who have not yet suffered a life-threatening arrhythmia yet remain at high risk of sudden cardiac death. The use of ICDs is justified as a "primary" preventative measure in these patients. One important group in this category comprises those patients with severe impairment of ventricular function after MI who have non-sustained VT on Holter monitoring and inducible VT on electrophysiological testing.

Another group of patients who may justify insertion of an ICD as a primary preventative strategy are those with inherited conditions associated with a high risk of sudden cardiac death. These include structural disorders of cardiac muscle as well as physiological disorders involving abnormal ion transport mechanisms in the cell membrane.

The photographs of the changes in ICDs over 10 years and the chest radiograph of the biventricular pacemaker are reproduced with permission from the chapter on 'Implantable devices for treating tachyarrythmias' by Timothy Houghton and Gerry C Kaye in the *ABC of Interventional Cardiology*. London: BMJ Publishing Group, 2004. The ICDs from 1992 and 2002 were supplied by C D Finlay, CRT coordinator, Guidant Canada Corporation, Toronto

---

ICDs for primary prevention

- Patients with severe impairment of ventricular function following MI
- Patients with inherited conditions linked with high risk of sudden cardiac death
- A history of MI plus
  Non sustained VT on 24 hour ECG monitoring
  Inductive VT on electrophysiological testing
  Left ventricular dysfunction with an ejection fraction of less than 35% but no worse than Class 3 of the New York Heart Association classification of heart failure
- Familial cardiac conditions with high risk of sudden death incuding:
  – long QT syndrome
  – hypertrophic cardiomyopathy
  – bugada syndrome
  – arrhythmogenic right ventricular dysplasia (AVRD)
  – after repair of Tetralogy of Fallot

The National Institute for Clinical Excellence (NICE) published guidance for the implantation of ICDs applicable to the United Kingdom in September 2000. These include recommendations for their use in patients who have been successfully resuscitated from cardiac arrest or who have sustained life-threatening arrhythmias

---

The results of the MADIT II trial are likely to widen the indications for the prophylactic use of ICDs. This study investigated whether implantation of an ICD would reduce mortality in high-risk patients with coronary disease and impaired left ventricular function. The trial, which had no arrhythmia entry criteria, was stopped prematurely after a 30% reduction in mortality was observed in post-MI patients with impaired left ventricular function randomised to receive an ICD

Further reading

- American College of Cardiology/American Heart Association. Guidelines for the implantation of cardiac pacemakers and antiarrhythmia devices. *JACC* 1998;31:1175-209.
- Coats AJ. MADIT II, the Multicentre Automatic Defibrillator Implantation Trial II stopped early for mortality reduction. Has ICD therapy earned its evidence-based credentials? *Int J Cardiol* 2002;82:1-5.
- Griffith MJ, Garratt CJ. Implantable devices for ventricular fibrillation and ventricular tachycardia. In: Julian DG, Camm AJ, Fox KM, Hall RJC, Poole-Wilson PA, eds. *Diseases of the heart.* 2nd ed. London: WB Saunders, 1996.
- National Institute for Clinical Excellence. Guidance on the use of implantable cardioverter defibrillators for arrhythmias. Technology appraisal guidance no 11. London: NICE, 2000.
- Kishore AGR, Camm AJ, Bennett DH. Cardiac pacing. In: Julian DG, Camm AJ, Fox KM, Hall RJC, Poole-Wilson PA, eds. *Diseases of the heart.* 2nd ed. London: WB Saunders, 1996.
- Klein H, Auricchio A, Reek S, Geller C. New primary prevention trials of sudden cardiac death in patients with left ventricular dysfunction: SCD-HeFT and MADIT II. *Am J Cardiol* 1999;83:91D-97D.

18   Infection risks and resuscitation

A J Harry Walmsley, David A Zideman

In cardiopulmonary resuscitation basic life support (airway, breathing, and circulation) should not be delayed regardless of whether the possible infective state of the patient has been established. A great deal has been written about the risk of contact of healthcare workers, rescuers, first aiders, and the general public with blood or body fluids of patients being resuscitated who are considered to be possible carriers of blood borne viruses (BBVs).

The potential risks of infection to the rescuer are from two sources: airway management (airway and breathing) and needlestick injuries (circulation).

Although BBVs are the greatest potential risk to rescuers, other non-viral organisms can pose a threat (tuberculosis and meningococcus). If mouth-to-mouth ventilation is performed on a patient with open tuberculosis then the rescuer is at risk. Follow up in a chest clinic, including checking BCG status, will be necessary. Contact with droplet spray from a patient infected with meningococcal disease will require the rescuer to receive prophylactic antibiotics.

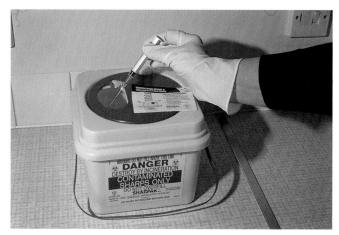

Sharps box

Guidelines

A report from the Centers for Disease Control has emphasised that blood is the single most important source of human immunodeficiency virus (HIV), and hepatitis B (HBV) and C (HCV) viruses through the parenteral, mucous membrane, or non-intact skin exposure. However, other high-risk body fluids, such as semen, vaginal secretions, and cerebrospinal, synovial, pleural, peritoneal, pericardial, and amniotic fluids, should have the same universal precautions applied. Low-risk body fluids to which these universal precautions are less important include saliva, sputum, nasal secretions, faeces, sweat, tears, urine, and vomit, unless they contain visible blood. A series of epidemiological studies of the non-sexual contacts of patients with HIV suggests that the possibility of salivary transmission of HIV is remote, and a further study has shown that hepatitis B was not transmitted from resuscitation manikins.

Risk from needlestick injuries

- Transmission of BBVs
  HBV
  HCV
  HIV
- Seroconversion from known positive donor
  30% HBV
  3% HCV
  0.3% HIV
  0.03% if contamination to eyes or mouth

Airway management

Wherever possible, healthcare workers and members of the general public should use some form of interpositional airway device when performing mouth-to-mouth resuscitation. This is particularly important when the risk is increased, such as when the saliva of trauma patients may be contaminated with blood. Face shields and pocket masks are two such airway devices. Before recommending such a device it is important to be satisfied that it will function effectively in its protective role and not interfere with the resuscitation techniques. Users must be properly trained and regularly tested. They should be properly informed about cleaning, sterilisation, and disposal and must be sure that the device is immediately available at all times when cardiopulmonary resuscitation may be necessary.

Best practice demands that standard precautions against the transmission of infection should be used at all hospital

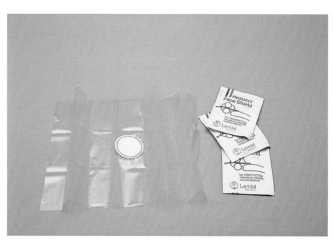

Face shield

resuscitation attempts. These should include face and eye protection and the use of gloves for both airway management and venous access.

Needlestick injuries

No evidence has been found to show that infection can be transmitted when the infected blood is in contact with intact skin.

In the United Kingdom, definitive seroconversion has been identified in only five healthcare workers who experienced percutaneous injuries when in contact with HIV-positive patients. Factors associated with an increased risk of HIV infection include deep injury, injury caused by visibly bloodstained devices, injury with a hollow bore needle that has been used in an artery or vein, and terminal HIV-related illness in the source patient. The risk of seroconversion after a single needlestick injury from a positive donor follows the "rule of 3s" (see box on p 87).

Action after exposure to HIV

A formal protocol of optimum management should exist in each Trust. Such management will normally be the responsibility of the Occupational Health Department, and a 24 hour Occupational Health Service should be routinely in place.

Post-exposure prophylaxis

The need for post-exposure prophylaxis (PEP) is determined by the risk of transmission and must be given as soon as possible. Triple therapy with anti-retroviral drugs virtually eliminates the risk of transmission. Both the United Kingdom and the United States recommend a four week course of triple therapy when the risk of exposure to HIV is high. The current recommended regime is zidovudine 300 mg and lamivudine 150 mg bd (Combivir) and nelfinavir 750 mg tds. An anti-emetic, such as domperidone, is often required. The most commonly reported side effects of these drugs are malaise, fatigue, insomnia, nausea, and vomiting.

Action after exposure to HBV and HCV

The greatest risk of acquiring a BBV infection from a needlestick injury comes from HBV E antigen positive, and surface antigen positive patients. If injury occurs, the recipient should have their antibody profile checked. High responders are at no risk. Low responders should receive a booster dose of vaccine and non-responders should receive HBV immunoglobulin; HBV transmission can be prevented if immunoglobulin is given within 48 hours.

The risk of acquiring HCV infection is small. However, at present no prophylactic measures are advised. If blood tests carried out between six and eight weeks after the potential infection are positive then antiviral treatment may be indicated.

Training manikins

Practice in resuscitation techniques is an essential part of establishing an effective resuscitation service. Resuscitation training manikins have not been shown to be sources of virus infection. Nevertheless, sensible precautions must be taken to minimise potential cross infection and the manikins must be formally disinfected after each use according to the manufacturers' recommendations.

Indications for post exposure prophylaxis (PEP)
- The donor is known or strongly suspected to be HIV positive
- The injury was deep
- The sharp was visibly bloodstained
- The injury was caused by a hollow bore needle that had been in an artery or vein
- Mucous membranes were exposed to body fluids or material at high risk of HIV infection

---

Advice on treatment for those who may have become infected
- Encourage skin puncture to bleed
- Wash liberally with soap and water
- Irrigate splashes into eyes or on mucous membrane with running water
- Report immediately to occupational health during working hours or to accident and emergency out of hours
- Complete accident or incident form
- Take 5-10 ml sample of clotted blood for hepatic and renal function
- Take blood sample for full blood count
- Take blood from the patient if fully informed consent is obtained
- Counselling, HIV testing, and drug prophylaxis may be required
- All information to be kept confidential

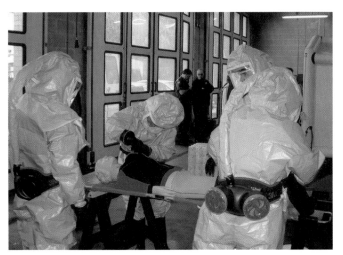

Biological or biochemical weapons decontamination practice

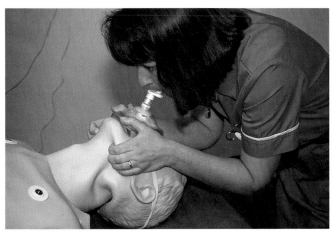

Using barrier methods to prevent contamination should be practised as manikins

Conclusion

Interpositional airway adjuncts should be used when performing mouth-to-mouth resuscitation. If a patient's oral cavity or saliva is contaminated with visible blood then the use of an adjunct can reassure the rescuer. However, as the risks of catching BBVs from rescue breathing are virtually nil (provided that blood is not present) then there must be no delay waiting for such an airway adjunct to be provided. In hospitals, standard precautions should be used routinely to minimise risk. Common sense and simple precautions will make the rescuer safe.

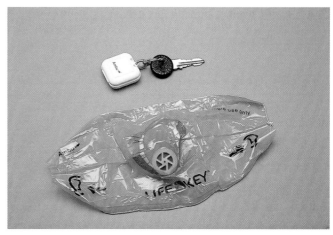

Life key

Further reading

- Cardo DM, Culver DH, Ciesielski CA, Srivastva PU, Marcus R, Abiteboul D, et al. Case control study of HIV seroconversion in health care workers after percutaneous exposure. *N Engl J Med* 1997;337:1485-90.
- Expert Advisory Group on AIDS, Advisory Group on Hepatitis. Guidance for clinical health care workers: protection against infection with blood borne viruses. Recommendations of the Expert Advisory Group on AIDS and the Advisory Group on Hepatitis [HSC 1998/063]. London: Department of Health, 1998.
- Henderson DK. Post exposure chemoprophylaxis for occupational exposures to the human immunodeficiency virus. *JAMA* 1999;281:931-6.
- Joint Committee on Vaccination and Immunisation. *Immunisation against infectious disease.* London: Department of Health, 1996.
- General Medical Council. *Serious communicable diseases.* London: General Medical Council, 1997.
- Taylor GP, Lyall BGH, Mercy D, Smith R, Chester T, Newall ML, et al. British HIV Association guidelines for prescribing anti-retroviral therapy in pregnancy. *Sex Transm Inf* 1999;75:96-7.

19 Teaching resuscitation

Ian Bullock, Geralyn Wynn, Carl Gwinnutt, Jerry Nolan, Sam Richmond, Jonathan Wylie, Bob Bingham, Michael Colquhoun, Anthony J Handley

Introduction

Education in resuscitation techniques has been a priority for many years in the United Kingdom, and the need to teach the necessary knowledge and skills remains a constant challenge. Increased awareness among the public of the possibility of successful resuscitation from cardiopulmonary arrest has added to the need to determine the best ways of teaching life-saving skills, both to healthcare professionals and to the general public. In the United Kingdom the Resuscitation Council (UK) has more than 10 years experience of running nationally accredited courses and these have established the benchmarks for best practice.

This chapter examines the principles of adult education and their application to the teaching of the knowledge and skills required to undertake resuscitation.

Levels of training

Resuscitation training may be categorised conveniently into four separate levels of attainment:

- Basic life support (BLS)
- BLS with airway adjuncts
- BLS with airway adjuncts plus defibrillation
- Advanced life support (ALS).

BLS
This comprises assessment of the patient, maintenance of the airway, provision of expired air ventilation, and support of the circulation by chest compression. It is essential that all healthcare staff who are in contact with patients are trained in BLS and receive regular updates with manikin practice. The general public should also be trained in the techniques.

BLS with airway adjuncts
The use of simple mechanical airways and devices that do not pass the oropharnyx is often included within the term BLS. The use of facemasks and shields should be taught to all healthcare workers. Increasingly, first-aiders and the general public also request training in the use of these aids.

BLS with airway adjuncts plus defibrillation
The use of defibrillators (whether automated or manual) should be taught to all hospital medical staff, especially trained nursing staff working in units in which cardiac arrest occurs often—for example, coronary care units, accident and emergency departments, and intensive therapy units—and to all emergency ambulance crews. Training should also be available to general practitioners, who should be encouraged to own defibrillators.

ALS
ALS techniques should be taught to all medical and nursing staff who may be required to provide definitive treatment for cardiac arrest patients. They may be members of the hospital resuscitation team or work in areas like the accident and emergency department or cardiac care unit, where cardiac

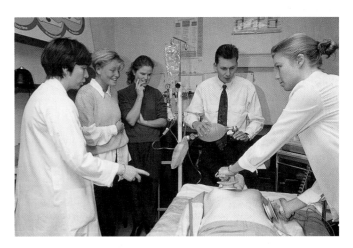

Medical students practising resuscitation

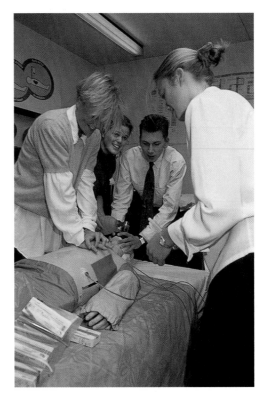

Medical students practising BLS and defibrillation

arrests occur most often. The techniques are taught to ambulance paramedics and to general practitioners who wish to acquire these skills.

Adults as learners

Most resuscitation training courses are designed for adults, and the educational process is very different to that used when teaching children. Adult candidates come to resuscitation courses from widely varying backgrounds and at different stages of their career development. Each individual has their own knowledge, strengths, anxieties, and hopes. Flexibility in the teaching of resuscitation will enable candidates to maximise their learning potential.

The previous knowledge and skills of an adult learner greatly influence their potential to acquire new knowledge and skills. Adults attending resuscitation courses have high intrinsic motivation because they recognise the potential application of what they are learning and how they can apply it to the everyday context.

The importance of being able to recognise the uniqueness of each candidate, and to create learning environments that help each individual, remains of the highest importance when teaching resuscitation techniques. This approach is largely accepted as an established principle in higher education and has had a substantial impact on how European resuscitation courses have developed.

The question of how medical personnel and others are trained to respond to cardiopulmonary arrest patients is a key issue, but high quality research into the best approach to teaching is lacking.

Although there seems to be a general acceptance that current training approaches are well developed and produce a high level of learner interaction, satisfaction, and professional development, little formal evaluation of courses has been reported to date.

Previous studies adopting an observational approach have shown the benefit of ALS training in improving the outcome from cardiac arrest. These studies are useful in providing information about the syllabus and conduct of training but fail to indicate the strengths and weaknesses of training classes, and it proves difficult to compare one approach with another.

Two important questions about the educational process are:

- How does it enable the acquisition of knowledge and skills and help their retention?
- How does it facilitate the maintenance of expertise and clinical effectiveness?

The process of learning is largely dependent on the individual and the preferred personal approach of that individual towards learning. In order to teach adults in an optimal fashion it is important to ensure that this individuality and preferred learning style is considered and provided for, wherever possible.

The importance of a balanced approach in delivering educational material means that no one of the four key areas of the curriculum (see box) is more important than the others. Yet many courses concentrate on only two of these areas, with the emphasis on knowledge and skills. Failing to acknowledge fully attitude and the building of relationships can have a detrimental effect on the outcome of this style of education.

Retention of resuscitation skills

This subject is one of the most studied areas of healthcare provision and several general principles have been established.

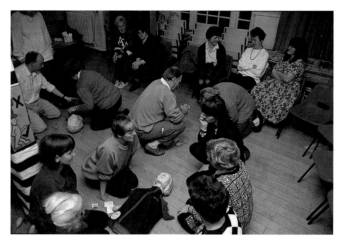
Group learning

Principles of adult education

- Adult learners are likely to be highly motivated
- They bring a wealth of experience to build upon
- Knowledge presented as relevant to their needs is more likely to be retained
- Timing a course to coincide with associated learning is likely to be most effective
- Instructors should be aware of the needs and expectations of the adult learner

Teaching adults

- Treat them as adults
- The "self" should not be under threat
- Ensure active participation and self evaluation as part of the process
- Previous experience should be recognised
- Include occupational requirements to heighten motivation

Key areas of the resuscitation curriculum

- Knowledge
- Skill
- Attitude
- Interpersonal relationships

The retention of both cognitive knowledge and psychomotor skills of cardiopulmonary resuscitation by healthcare professionals and the lay public declines rapidly and is substantially weaker four to six months after instruction. Individuals formally tested one year after training often show a level of skill similar to that before training. The degree of skill retention does not correlate with the thoroughness of the initial training. Even when candidates are assessed as being fully competent at the end of a training session the skill decay is still rapid. Neither doctors, nurses, nor the lay public can accurately predict their level of knowledge or skill at basic resuscitation techniques when compared with the results of formal evaluation.

Simplification of the training programme and the repetition of teaching and practice are the only techniques that have been shown to maximise recall. Research shows that experience acquired by attending actual cardiac arrests does not improve theoretical knowledge or skill in performing resuscitation. It has been shown that a health professional's confidence in performing resuscitation correlates poorly with their competence.

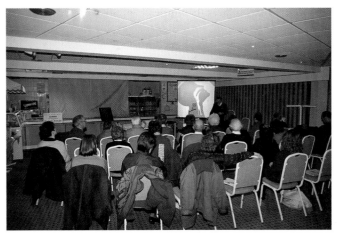

Adult BLS class

Teaching resuscitation skills

Resuscitation uses skills that are essentially practical, and practical training is necessary to acquire them; the development of sophisticated training manikins and other teaching aids has greatly assisted this process. Repetition of both theory and practice is an important component of any training programme.

Role-play or simulation is used extensively to allow the candidate to incorporate new information into their own real world. The use of visual imagery to integrate skills acquired is one that healthcare professionals seem to be comfortable with and it adds a dynamic element. It also allows the candidate to apply the abstract components of new knowledge into the real world of everyday work. Asking candidates to think about clinical situations they have experienced will help them to appreciate their previous knowledge and allow the teacher to base new learning around this.

The mastery of skills is concerned with how the candidate interacts with the teaching environment and is shaped by previous knowledge, skill, and attitude.

The process of acquiring new skills, and therefore changing behaviour, seems to be dependent on the candidates being able to relate the new learning to their immediate situation. It is this "situation dependency" that enables candidates to organise, process, and apply new learning successfully into their work. Put simply, the educational approach is linked to their real world. Opportunities for candidates to integrate new knowledge, skills, and attitudes into their everyday practice need to be shaped as structured learning opportunities. These are constructed in a four-stage approach.

The four-stage teaching approach

This represents a staged approach to teaching a skill that is designed to apply the principles of adult learning to the classroom. The process is about knowledge and skill transference from an expert instructor to that of a novice (a candidate who aspires to be a member of the cardiac arrest team). In the staged approach the responsibility for performing the skill is gradually placed further away from the instructor and closer to the learner. The goal is a change in behaviour, with performance enhanced through regular practice.

Retention of resuscitation skills

- Poor retention in healthcare professionals and lay people evaluated from two weeks to three years after training
- Individuals tested one year after training often show skills similar to those before training
- Healthcare professionals and lay people cannot accurately predict their level of knowledge or skill at basic techniques
- The degree of skill retention does not correlate with the thoroughness of the training
- Simplification of the programme and repetition are the only techniques to have demonstrated recall
- Repeated refresher courses have been shown to help retention of psychomotor skills
- No evidence to show attendance at a cardiac arrest improves retention of knowledge or skills
- Healthcare professionals' confidence in their resuscitation skills correlates poorly with their ability

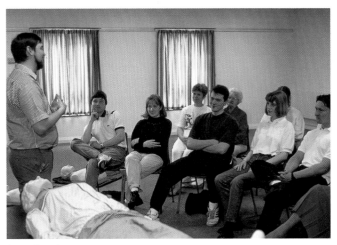

Group learning

This approach places the emphasis on the candidate's ability to frame learning around recognisable scenarios and removes the abstract thought necessary to acquire skills in isolation.

Training healthcare workers

Resuscitation Council (UK) training courses

Practical training is an essential component of all the ALS courses developed by the Resuscitation Council (UK). These cover the resuscitation of both adult (ALS) and paediatric subjects (PALS) and have become widely available during the past 10 years. A neonatal life support course (NLS) was introduced in 2001. In order that the resuscitation courses administered by the Resuscitation Council (UK) are based on good educational practice, the Generic Instructor Course was developed. All potential instructors attend this course. The focus is to develop the ability to teach the related core skills of resuscitation within a universal approach to teaching.

The ALS course

In the United Kingdom, training in resuscitation before 1990 was sporadic and uncoordinated. A study in 1981 found that in a group of junior hospital doctors tested none were able to perform BLS to American Heart Association standards. By the mid 1980s little had changed; although over half the junior doctors tested could attempt BLS, the standard to which it was being performed was just as poor. Similar results were reported among nursing staff. In response to these findings, the Royal College of Physicians recommended that all doctors, medical students, nurses, dental practitioners, and paramedical staff should undergo regular training in the management of cardiopulmonary arrest.

As a direct response, the first British course was held the same year at St Bartholomew's Hospital, London, using Resuscitation Council (UK) guidelines. Over the following five years, ALS-type courses were set up in a variety of centres throughout the United Kingdom and by 1994 a standardised ALS course was established under the direction of the Resuscitation Council (UK). The aim of the course was "to teach the theory and practical skills required to manage cardiopulmonary arrest in an adult from the time when arrest seems imminent, until either the successful resuscitation of the patient who enters the Intensive or Cardiac Care Unit, or the resuscitation attempt is abandoned and the patient declared dead."

The ALS course was originally designed to be appropriate for all healthcare professionals working in a clinical environment. All participants, whatever their background or grade, are taught using standardised material and the latest European Resuscitation Council (ERC) guidelines and algorithms. For each course, the programme and participating instructors must be registered and approved by the Resuscitation Council (UK). Quality control is reinforced by evaluation forms completed by the candidates and by the use of regional representatives who are empowered to visit and inspect courses and provide independent feedback.

The course is very intensive and lasts a minimum of two days, with a maximum candidate-to-faculty ratio of 3:1. The multidisciplinary faculty must be ALS instructors or instructor candidates (those who have completed the instructor course but have yet to complete two teaching assignments). All candidates receive the ALS course manual at least four weeks before attending the course, together with a multiple choice test for self-assessment, and are expected to be competent in BLS. During the course, a series of practical skill

The four-stage teaching approach

Stage 1: silent demonstration of the skill
In this first stage, the instructor demonstrates the skill as normally undertaken, without any commentary or explanation. The procedure is performed at the normal speed to achieve realism and thereby help the student to absorb the instructor's expertise. It allows the learner a unique "fly on the wall" insight into the performance of the skill. Through the instructor's demonstration the candidate has a benchmark of excellence, an animated performance that will facilitate the acquirement of the skill, and help move him or her from novice to expert

Stage 2: repeat demonstration with dialogue informing learners of the rationale for actions
This stage allows the transference of factual information from teacher to learner. Here, the instructor is able to slow down the whole performance of the skill, explain the basis for his actions, and, where appropriate, indicate the evidence base for the skill. During this stage the instructor leads candidates from what they already know to what they need to know. The opportunity to reinforce important principles helps to facilitate the integration of information and psychomotor skills. Importantly, the learner is engaged and involved in the practice of the skill, without being threatened by the need to perform it

Stage 3: repeat demonstration guided by one of the learners
The responsibility for performing the skill now firmly moves towards the learner, with emphasis on using cognitive understanding to guide the psychomotor activity. The learner talks the instructor through the skill in a staged and logical sequence based on recollection of the previously observed practice. It is also the responsibility of the instructor to ensure that, in simulated practice, the skill is not seen in relative isolation but is placed within the proper context of a real cardiac arrest. Time to reflect on the skill learnt and the opportunity to ask questions all add to the importance of this stage, and positive reinforcement of good practice by the instructor helps to shape the future practice of the individual learner

Stage 4: repeat demonstration by the learner and practice of the skill by all learners
This stage completes the teaching and learning process, and helps establish the ability of the student to perform a particular skill. It is this stage that the skills are transferred from the expert (instructor) to the novice (candidate), with the candidate being an active investigator of the environment rather than a passive recipient of stimuli and rewards

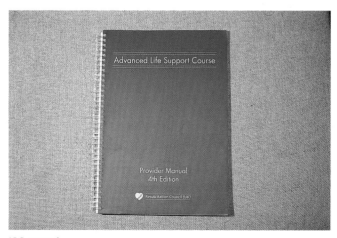

ALS manual

stations and workshops, supplemented by lectures, are used to teach airway management, defibrillation, arrhythmia recognition, the use of drugs, and post-resuscitation care. Causes and prevention of cardiac arrest, cardiac arrest in special circumstances, ethical issues, and the management of bereavement are also covered.

The overall emphasis of the course is towards the team management of cardiac arrest. This is taught in cardiac arrest simulation (CASteach) scenarios that are designed to be as realistic as possible, using modern manikins and up-to-date resuscitation equipment. Each scenario is designed to allow the candidates to integrate the knowledge and skills learnt while, at the same time, developing the interpersonal skills required for team leadership. During the course, summative assessments are made of the candidates' abilities to perform BLS, airway control, and defibrillation. A further multiple choice paper, which includes questions on rhythm recognition, is undertaken. Finally, overall skills are assessed using a cardiac arrest simulation test (CAStest). Standardised test scenarios and uniform assessment criteria are used to ensure that every candidate (independent of course centre) reaches the same national standard.

Successful candidates receive a Resuscitation Council (UK) ALS Provider Certificate, valid for three years, after which they are encouraged to undertake a recertification course to ensure that they remain up-to-date. The award of this certificate only implies successful completion of the course and does not constitute a licence to practise the skills taught. Participants who show the appropriate qualities to be an instructor are invited to attend a two day Generic Instructor Course, supervised by an educationalist, which focuses on lecturing techniques and the teaching of practical skills.

PALS course

PALS courses follow similar principles to those for adults. They last two days, are multidisciplinary, and encourage the development of teamwork. The majority of the training is carried out in small groups, and scenarios are used throughout. At the end an assessment is carried out, which is based on basic and ALS scenarios and a multiple choice questionnaire.

PALS is an international course that was initially developed by the American Heart Association and the American Academy of Pediatrics in the late 1980s. It was introduced into Europe and the United Kingdom in 1992 and is run in the United Kingdom under the auspices of the Resuscitation Council (UK) using ERC guidelines. This has allowed the regulations for PALS courses to mirror those for ALS (see above) and for the Council to ensure that standards remain high.

Since 1992 there has been rapid expansion; in the first five years over 5000 providers were trained and 540 instructors now teach at 48 course centres. Instructors are selected for their experience with acutely ill children, their ability to communicate, and their performance during the provider course. After selection they undertake the Generic Instructor Course followed by a period of supervised teaching until they are considered to be fully trained.

The ERC is currently developing its own PALS course that will be similar in content and format to the American Heart Association version. It is planned that this will eventually replace PALS in the United Kingdom. It is also planned that instructor and provider qualifications will be fully transferable from PALS (UK) to the European course.

Newborn life support course

Resuscitation at birth is needed in around 10% of all deliveries in the United Kingdom. Thus, it is the most common form of

By the end of 2001, over 65 000 healthcare professionals had successfully completed a Resuscitation Council (UK) ALS Course. The ALS course is now well established throughout the United Kingdom, with about 550 courses being run annually in over 200 centres. After the 1998 guidelines update, the course manual was adopted by the ERC as the core material for a European ALS course. The fourth edition of the ALS manual was published in 2000 and incorporated recommendations made in the International Guidelines 2000 for Cardiopulmonary Resuscitation. The ALS manual has been translated into Portuguese, Italian, and German and the ALS course has now been adopted by 11 countries across Europe

The great advantage of a multidisciplinary ALS course is that the doctors, nurses, and other healthcare professionals who will be working together as a resuscitation team, train and practise together. This contributes to the realism of simulation and encourages constructive interaction between team members. However, not all healthcare staff require a comprehensive ALS course; they may be overwhelmed with information and skills that are not relevant to their practice and this will distract them from acquiring the core skills. In an attempt to meet the needs of these healthcare providers and standardise much of the training already undertaken by Resuscitation Officers, the Resuscitation Council (UK) has introduced a one-day Immediate Life Support (ILS) course at the beginning of 2002. This course provides certified training in prevention of cardiac arrest, BLS, safe defibrillation, airway management with basic adjuncts, and cardiac arrest team membership

The PALS course is multidisciplinary: 50% of the participants are medical and 50% come from nursing, paramedical, or allied professions. Although suitable for anyone who may encounter sick children, the course is aimed particularly at doctors training in specialties involving the care of children, and nurses and allied healthcare workers specialising in acute or emergency paediatrics

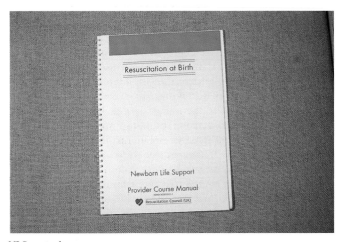

NLS manual

resuscitation. The outcome is usually successful; 95% of resuscitated newborns survive and 95% of the survivors are normal. The need for resuscitation at birth is only partly predictable: 50% of all resuscitation takes place after an apparently normal pregnancy and labour. This means that all professionals who may be involved with deliveries—for example, midwives, paediatricians, neonatal nurses, obstetricians, anaesthetists, and ambulance personnel—need training in resuscitation of the newborn.

The material taught is consistent with current European and International Guidelines and is published as the *Resuscitation at Birth—The Newborn Life Support Provider Course Manual*. This has been produced by a multidisciplinary committee working under the auspices of the Resuscitation Council (UK). The theoretical and practical skills taught include the following:

- The provision of the right environment and temperature control
- Airway management using mask techniques
- Chest compression
- Vascular access and the use of resuscitation drugs.

The course then moves beyond the acquisition of basic skills to scenarios using manikins to simulate various types of resuscitation so that candidates can put the techniques learnt into practice. Candidates are assessed during the course and guidance is provided by a mentoring system so that problems can be rectified in good time. Candidates are tested at the end of the course by multiple-choice questions and a practical airway test in the form of a structured scenario or OSCI.

The course was formally launched by the Resuscitation Council (UK) in April 2001 with support from the medical Royal Colleges and professional bodies like the British Association of Perinatal Medicine. Since the launch of this course, 30 course centres have been approved and nearly 100 provider courses have been held, 130 instructors have been fully trained, and a further 97 are undertaking the GIC course. Nearly 2500 providers have been trained, of whom nearly 40% are either midwives or nurses. The interest expressed by large numbers of professionals working with the newborn indicates that the NLS course will follow other Resuscitation Council (UK) courses in training large numbers of providers and thereby improving practice in the resuscitation of the newborn in the United Kingdom.

Training the public

Campaigns to teach BLS to members of the public in the United Kingdom have gained momentum in the 1990s as front-line ambulances became equipped with defibrillators. Training in BLS is provided by the voluntary first aid societies and the Royal Life Saving Society (UK). Pioneering schemes to teach the public have become increasingly common in recent years and many are coordinated through the Heartstart (UK) initiative of the British Heart Foundation. This scheme has a facilitatory role as well as providing practical help and financial support through professional coordinators and back-up staff. To date, more than 700 separate community-based schemes have become affiliated to Heartstart (UK). Each one aims to teach BLS to the lay public in a single session lasting about two hours. Instruction on the treatment of choking and the recovery position is also usually included. The basic syllabus is covered in the booklet *Resuscitation for the Citizen*, published by the Resuscitation Council (UK). The Foundation has also produced a range of teaching aids, such as booklets, wall charts,

Newborn resuscitation

- Teaching neonatal resuscitation has traditionally been carried out informally in the delivery room. This approach is flawed because it cannot reach all the disciplines that need to acquire these skills, it does not allow time to practise skills like correct mask ventilation, and it leads to the haphazard passing on of both good and bad practice. Structured teaching, which has been so successful in improving resuscitation practice for older patients, is now being applied to the newborn
- The Resuscitation Council (UK) has developed a multidisciplinary NLS course in line with its other ALS courses. This course is based on the same educational principles. The emphasis is on a firm understanding of the underlying physiology, followed by the learning of individual skills, and then the integration of the two into scenarios that promote working with other professionals in a team. Instructors are professionals with ongoing responsibility for providing resuscitation at birth who have shown exceptional ability while attending the provider course. They will then be required to undergo further training in how to teach by attending the Generic Instructor Course

Useful addresses

- The British Heart Foundation
  14 Fitzhardinge Street
  London W1H 4DH
- The Resuscitation Council (UK)
  5th floor
  Tavistock House North
  London WC1H 9JR
- The British Red Cross Society
  9 Grosvenor Crescent
  London SW1X 7EJ
- The Royal Life Saving Society UK
  River House
  High Street
  Broom
  Warwickshire B50 4HN
- St Andrew's Ambulance Association
  St Andrew's House
  48 Milton Street
  Glasgow G4 0HR
- St John Ambulance
  27 St John's Lane
  London EC1M 4BU

Several studies have clearly shown the value of BLS initiated by bystanders before the arrival of the emergency medical services

Schools

The teaching of first aid is not universal in British schools nor is knowledge of first aid required of every teacher. The subject is included within the National Curriculum in England and Wales but it is not compulsory. By contrast, BLS skills have been taught regularly in schools in other European countries, most notably Norway, for almost 40 years and successful application of the techniques has been reported. In recent years, the British Heart Foundation has promoted the teaching of BLS skills in schools through its Heartstart (UK) initiative. Individual schools are able to affiliate to the scheme and receive specially developed training materials and financial help towards the purchase of training manikins videos, and a variety of other support materials. Trainers are recruited from the statutory ambulance service and the voluntary first aid and life saving societies; many schemes have trained their own instructors. Practising the techniques on training manikins is an essential part of these classes and enforces the theoretical instruction provided.

Conclusion

The problem is to discover the best way to ensure that resuscitation skills are well taught, well learnt, and well retained. Much effort has been put into the development of training courses for lay people as well as healthcare professionals, and this does result in higher skill levels. Much work is still needed to address the problem of the rapid loss of knowledge and ability seen in all groups of learners. Good teaching, plenty of "hands-on" practice, and frequent retraining all seem to help. Ultimately, the real solution may lie in simplifying the techniques that are taught.

Further reading

- Resuscitation Council (UK). *Cardiopulmonary Resuscitation: Guidance for practice and training for hospitals.* London: Resuscitation Council (UK), 2000.
- Resuscitation Council (UK). *Cardiopulmonary Resuscitation: Guidance for practice and training for primary care.* London: Resuscitation Council (UK), 2001.
- Eisenberg M, Bergner L, Hallstron A. Cardiac resuscitation in the community. Importance of rapid provision and implications for programme planning. *JAMA* 1979;241:190.
- Martean TM, Wynne G, Kaye W, Evans TR Resuscitation: Experience without feedback increases confidence but not skill. *BMJ* 1990;300:849-50.
- Kaye W, Mancini ME, Rallis SF. *Educational aspects: resuscitation training and evaluation. Clinics in critical care medicine.* Edinburgh: Churchill Livingstone, 1989.
- Knowles MS. *The adult learner—a neglected species.* London: Houston Publishing Company, 1984.
- Lowenstein SR. CPR by medical and surgical house officers. *Lancet* 1981;ii:679.
- Skinner D. CPR skills of preregistration house officers. *BMJ* 1985;290:1549.
- Wynne GA. Inability of trained nurses to perform basic life support. *BMJ* 1987;294:1198.
- Royal College of Paediatrics and Child Health, Royal College of Obstetrics and Gynaecologists. *Resuscitation of babies at birth.* London: BMJ Books, 1997.
- Royal College of Physicians. Resuscitation from cardiopulmonary arrest: training and organisation. *J R Coll Physicians Lond* 1987;21:1.
- Working Group of the European Resuscitation Council. Recommendations on resuscitation of babies at birth. *Resuscitation* 1998;37:103-10.

20 Training manikins

Gavin D Perkins, Michael Colquhoun, Robert Simons

Both theoretical and practical skills are required to perform cardiopulmonary resuscitation. Theoretical skills can be learnt in the classroom, from written material or computer programmes. The acquisition of practical skills, however, requires the use of training manikins. It is impracticable as well as potentially dangerous to practise these procedures on human volunteers.

Adult and paediatric manikins are available from several manufacturers worldwide; this chapter concentrates on those generally available in the United Kingdom.

Manikin selection: general principles

Training requirements

The growing number of different manikins available today can make choosing which manikin to purchase a complex process. The most important question to ask initially is: which skills need to be acquired? This will obviously depend on the class under instruction; the requirements of a lay class will be quite different from those of professional hospital staff learning advanced life support skills. The size of the class will also be important. For large classes it may be better to maximise the practical hands-on exposure by investing in several cheaper manikins rather than rely on one or two expensive, more complex models.

Visual display and recording

Manikins differ in the amount of feedback that they give to both student and instructor and in their ability to provide details about performance. Models vary greatly in sophistication, but most provide some qualitative indication that technique is adequate, such as audible clicks when the depth of chest compression is correct. Some manikins incorporate sensors that recognise the correct hand position and the rescuer's attempts at shaking, opening the airway, and palpation of a pulse. The depths of ventilation and chest compression may also be recorded. An objective assessment of performance may be communicated to the student or instructor by means of flashing lights, meters, audible signals, or graphical display on a screen. A permanent record may be obtained for subsequent study or certification.

Manikins that interface with computers will measure performance for a set period and compare adequacy of technique against established standards, such as those of the European Resuscitation Council or the American Heart Association. A score, indicating the number of correct manoeuvres, may form the basis of a test of competence. However, the software algorithms in some assessment programmes are very strict and only minimal deviations from these standards is tolerated. A minimum score of 70% correct cardiac compressions and ventilations may be taken to represent effective life support. This score on a Skillmeter Resusci Anne manikin is acceptable to the Royal College of General Practitioners of the United Kingdom as part of the MRCGP examination.

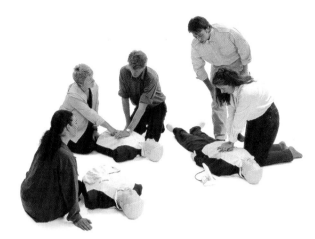

Manikins are vital for learning practical cardiopulmonary resuscitation skills

> With all manikins, realistic appearance, accurate anatomical landmarks, and an appropriate response to any attempted resuscitation manoeuvre are essential

---

Resuscitation skills that can be practised on manikins

Basic life support
- Manual airway control with or without simple airway adjuncts
- Pulse detection
- Expired air ventilation (mouth-to-mouth or mouth-to-mask)
- Chest compression
- Treatment of choking
- Automated external defibrillation

Advanced techniques
- Precordial thump
- Airway management skills
- Interpretation of electrocardiographic arrhythmia
- Defibrillation and cardioversion
- Intravenous and intraosseous access (with or without administration of drugs)

Related skills
- Management of haemorrhage, fractures, etc.
- Treatment of pneumothorax
- Nursing care skills

Maintenance and repair

Manikins should be easy to clean. Some care is required, however, and the "skin" should not be permanently marked by lipstick or pens or allowed to become stained with extensive use. Many currently available manikins have replacements available for those components subject to extensive wear and tear. This is particularly true for the face, which bears the brunt of damage and where discoloration or wear will make the manikin aesthetically unattractive.

Manikins are bulky and require adequate space for storage. A carrying case (preferably rigid and fitted with castors for heavier manikins) is essential for safe storage and transport.

Cross infection and safety

To minimise the risk of infection occurring during the conduct of simulated mouth-to-mouth ventilation the numbers of students using each manikin should be kept low and careful attention should be paid to hygiene. Students should be free of communicable infection, particularly of the face, mouth, or respiratory tract. Faceshields or other barrier devices (see Chapter 18) should be used when appropriate. Manikins should be disinfected during and after each training session according to the manufacturer's instructions. Preparations incorporating 70% alcohol and chlorhexidine are often used. Hypochlorite solutions containing 500 ppm chlorine (prepared by adding 20 ml of domestic bleach to 1 l of water) are effective but unpleasant to use. They are best reserved for the thorough cleaning of manikins between classes. Moulded hair has now replaced stranded or artificial hair and is much easier to keep clean.

Many modern manikins feature a disposable lower airway consisting of plastic lungs and connecting tubes. Expired air passes through a non-return valve in the side of the manikin during expiration. All disposable parts should be replaced in accordance with the manufacturer's recommendations. Other manikins use a clean mouthpiece and disposable plastic bag insert for each student.

Cost

Cost will depend on the skills to be practised and the number of manikins required for a class. Sophisticated skills, such as monitoring, recording, and reporting facilities, increase cost further. Any budget should include an allowance for cleaning, provision of disposable items, and replacement parts. Another consideration is the ease with which the manikins can be updated when resuscitation guidelines and protocols change.

Manikins for basic life support

Airway

The ability to open the airway by tilting the head or lifting the jaw, or both, is a feature of practically all manikins currently available. Modern manikins cannot be ventilated unless the appropriate steps to secure a patent airway have been taken.

Regrettably, some manikins require excessive neck extension to secure airway patency; such action would be quite inappropriate in the presence of an unstable injury to the cervical spine.

Back blows and abdominal thrusts used to treat the choking casualty can be practised convincingly only on a manikin made specifically for that purpose. A degree of simulation is, however, possible with most manikins.

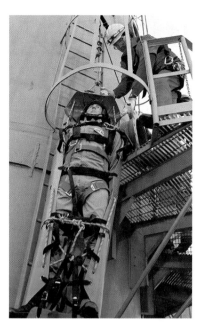

Manikins can be used for a variety of training exercises

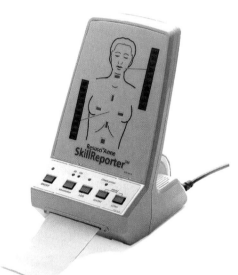

Some manikins produce printed reports on performance

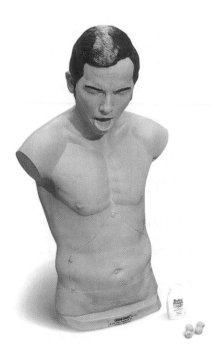

Choking Charlie can be used for the simulation of the management of choking

Breathing

Most currently available manikins offer realistic simulation of chest wall compliance and resistance to expired air ventilation. In some manikins attempts to inflate the chest when the airway is inadequately opened or the use of excessive ventilation pressure will result in distension of the "stomach." Some advanced manikins feature a stomach bag that may be emptied by the instructor under appropriate circumstances and used to simulate regurgitation into the patient's mouth.

Mouth-to-nose ventilation is difficult to perform on some manikins because the nose is small, too soft, too hard, or has inadequate nostrils. Access for nasal catheters and airways is also impracticable on most manikins for this reason.

The design of most basic manikins does not readily permit the use of simple airway adjuncts—for example, the Guedel airway—because space in the oropharynx and hypopharynx is limited; special airway trainers are more suitable. The quality of ventilation while using a facemask depends on the seal between the mask and face of the manikin; a mask with an inflatable cuff will provide a better contact and seal. Similar considerations apply when a bag-valve-mask device is used. The rather rigid and inflexible faces of most manikins dictate that a firm, one-handed grip is required to prevent air leaks; in real life, a two-handed grip may be required on such occasions.

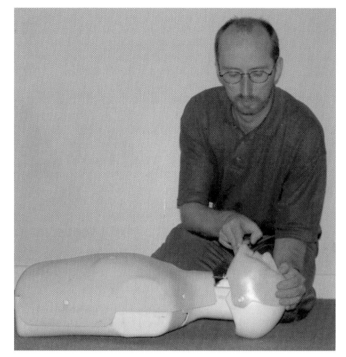

Opening the airway

Circulation

The value of the pulse check to confirm cardiac arrest has recently been challenged. Although several manikins can generate, a palpable pulse (electronically or manually by squeezing an air bulb attached to the manikin by plastic tubing) this is becoming less important, especially for lay rescuers.

Chest compression should be practised on manikins with appropriate chest wall compliance and recoil. Many manikins give some form of indication that the depth of compression is adequate, and some monitor the hand position. Few, if any, manikins allow carotid pulsation to be activated by rescuer chest compression.

Defibrillation

The use of automated external defibrillators (AEDs) is now considered to be part of the repertoire of basic life support skills. Some manufacturers produce training AEDs or models with separate training modules that generate a number of different scenarios for practice. These training AEDs cannot generate an electric countershock and so may be safely used with a standard basic life support manikin by attaching the training electrodes to the manikin's chest. However, if a fully functional AED is used for training it is imperative that a manikin is used that has been specifically designed for defibrillation practice; it is dangerous to discharge the shock onto a standard manikin. Manikins for AED training either offer a number of pre-determined scenarios or allow the operator to determine his or her own scenarios. In addition to selecting the underlying rhythm, the operator may be able to prompt the defibrillator to give warnings such as "check pads position" or "call engineer." Most advanced life support manikins that allow manual defibrillation will also allow defibrillation with an AED provided that the correct leads connecting the two machines are available. Before using a manikin for AED training it is important to refer to the manufacturer's instructions to ensure that the AED and manikin are compatible.

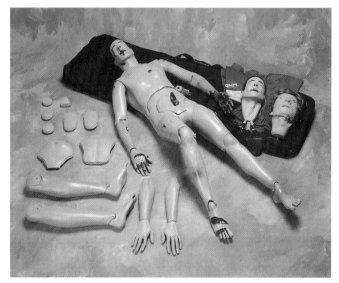

Crash Kelly—some manikins can be used for trauma scenarios

The recovery position

Practising the recovery position is impracticable with manikins lacking flexible bodies and jointed limbs; in most cases a human volunteer is needed.

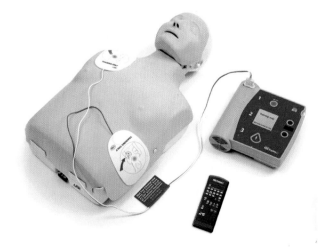

Laerdal AED training system

Manikins for advanced life support

Manikins for advanced life support training should ideally allow multiple tasks to be undertaken concurrently—for example, basic life support, electrocardiographic monitoring, defibrillation, tracheal intubation, and intravenous cannulation—and interaction or control of the scenario by the instructor. This enables team management of a cardiac arrest to be practised in an interactive fashion with the instructor altering conditions and presenting an evolving scenario in response to the treatment given.

Some manikins feature optional extras that allow simulation of a variety of injuries—for example, burns, lacerations, and fractures. Other models permit procedures such as transtracheal jet ventilation, cricothyrotomy, pericardiocentesis, surgical venous access, and tube thoracostomy. Features such as these have proved invaluable for training in trauma care.

Airway management

Manikins dedicated to the teaching of airway management feature a head and neck containing an accurate simulation of the anatomy of the oropharynx and larynx. These models are usually mounted on a rigid baseboard that ensures stability while the head and neck are manoeuvred. Infant and neonatal equivalents are also available.

A range of airway adjuncts may be used, although not all manikins allow practice of the full repertoire. In addition to the static airway manikins, a recent addition to the market allows the instructor to make dynamic changes to the condition of the airway. Through a complex set of inflatable bladders built into the manikin, it is possible to simulate trismus, laryngospasm, tongue swelling, pharyngeal obstruction, tension pneumothorax, and complete airway obstruction. In this way trainees can experience diverse and changing airway problems within the safe environment of a simulation exercise.

Careful choice of a robust airway management trainer is recommended, and a lubricant spray or jelly should always be used. Damage to the mouth, tongue, epiglottis, and larynx is common so it is important to be sure that repair or replacement of these parts is easy and relatively inexpensive.

Breathing

Most manikins respond to artificial ventilation by symmetrical chest movement. Incorrect intubation, such as tube placement in the right main bronchus or oesophagus, will result in unilateral chest movement or distension of the stomach, respectively. More complex manikins allow the instructor to control chest movements and can generate a variety of different breath sounds. In addition, some allow the simulation and treatment of a tension pneumothorax by needle thoracocentesis and chest drain insertion.

Electrocardiographic monitoring and rhythm recognition

The ability to monitor and interpret the cardiac rhythm is crucial to the management of cardiac emergencies. An electronic rhythm generator may be connected to suitably designed manikins to enable arrhythmias to be simulated. The digitised electrocardiographic signal from the device may be monitored through chest electrodes or from the manikin chest studs that are used for defibrillation. Basic models provide the minimum requirements of sinus rhythm and the rhythms responsible for cardiac arrest (ventricular fibrillation, ventricular tachycardia, and asystole). More advanced models provide a wide range of arrhythmias and the heart rate, rhythm, or QRST morphology may be changed instantly by the instructor. These devices may be programmed to change

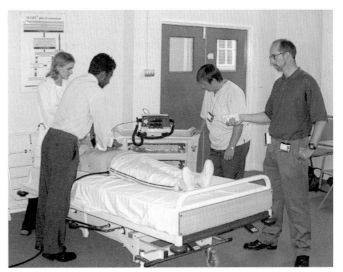
Manikin being used for advanced life support practice

It is vital for all personnel involved in the care of the acutely ill patient to be able to manage an airway

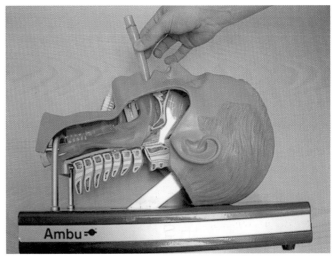
Ambu airway trainer shows cross-sectional anatomy of the airway

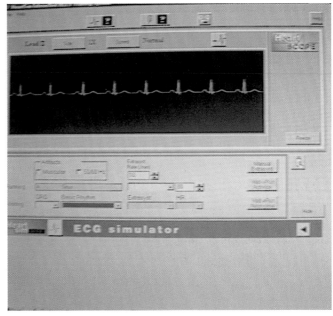
Electrocardiogram simulator

rhythm after the delivery of a direct current shock so that students are able to monitor the effects of defibrillation in a lifelike way. It should be remembered that energy levels of 50-400 J are potentially lethal, and a specially designed manikin defibrillation skin that incorporates an attenuator box must always be used.

Greater realism is provided by some manikins that produce a palpable pulse (and some blood pressure) when the electrocardiographic rhythm changes to one that is consistent with a cardiac output.

Intravenous access

Several models currently available enable practice in peripheral or central venous cannulation. A plastic skin overlies the "veins," which are simulated by plastic tubes containing coloured liquid. The skin provides a realistic impression of cutaneous resistance while the veins provide further resistance to the needle; once the vein is entered the coloured fluid can be aspirated. Some models allow the placement of intravenous catheters by the Seldinger or catheter-through-cannula technique. Some are available that allow peripheral venous cannulation in several different sites. Manikins for central venous cannulation allow access to the subclavian, jugular, and femoral veins; these feature appropriate anatomical landmarks and may incorporate a compressible bulb that enables the instructor to simulate adjacent arterial pulsation. Other models allow venous cut-down procedures to be performed. Some paediatric manikins allow the practise of intraosseous needle insertion, peripheral cannulation, scalp vein cannulation, and umbilical cord catheterisation.

Patient simulators

Patient simulators are a natural progression from advanced life support training manikins. They were developed initially for training anaesthetists and they are now used for a wide variety of different scenarios. At present, four medical simulation centres in the United Kingdom provide training courses in the management of a variety of clinical scenarios. The simulators are set up in a mock operating theatre, resuscitation room, or other clinical area, and participants are able to manage a simulated patient scenario and see instantly the results of their decisions and actions. The use of actual medical equipment allows participants to learn the advantages and limitations of different instruments and devices. Full physiological monitoring—for example, blood pressure, central venous pressure, cardiac output, 12 lead electrocardiogram, electroencephalogram, pupil size—can be controlled by the instructor, allowing an almost real life experience without any risk to patients or participants. A recent exciting development is the production of a portable patient simulator. Although not possessing all of the features described above, it offers considerable advantages in terms of cost, portability, and ease of use.

Conclusion

Important advances have been made in the development of manikins for resuscitation training in the past few years. A wide choice of different manikins (and prices) now allows a variety of skills and patient scenarios to be practised. Before making a decision to purchase such equipment it is important to be clear who and how many are to be trained, and what skills are to be taught.

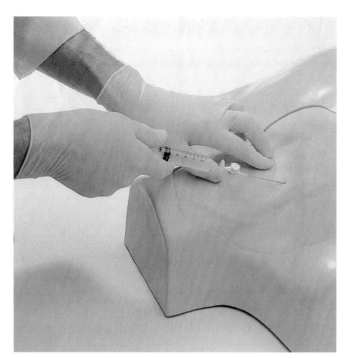

Laerdal intravenous torso can be used for central venous cannulation

Manufacturers and distributors

- Adam Rouilly (London) Ltd
  Crown Road
  Eurolink Business Park
  Sittingbourne
  Kent ME10 3AG
  Telephone: 01795 471378
  Fax: 01795 479787
- Drager Medical
  The Willows
  Mark Road,
  Hemel Hempstead
  Hertfordshire
  HP2 7BW
  Telephone: 01442 213542
  Fax: 01442 240327
- Laerdal Medical Ltd
  Laerdal House
  Goodmead Road
  Orpington,
  Kent BR6 0HX
  Telephone: 01689 876634
  Fax: 01689 873800
- Medicotest UK (Ambu)
  Burrel Road
  St Ives,
  Cambridgeshire PE27 3LE
  Telephone: 01480 498403
  Fax: 01480 498405

Further reading

- Committee for Evaluation of Sanitary Practices in CPR Training. Recommendations for decontaminating manikins used in CPR training. *Respiratory Care* 1984;29:1250-2.
- Issengerg SB, McGaghie WC, Hart IR, Mayer JW, Felner JM, Petrusa ER, et al. Simulation technology for health care professional skills training and assessment. *JAMA* 1999;282:861-6.
- Simons RS. Training aids and models. In Baskett PJF, ed. *Cardiopulmonary resuscitation.* Amsterdam: Elsevier, 1989.

21 The ethics of resuscitation

Peter J F Baskett

Present-day knowledge, skill, pharmacy, and technology have proved effective in prolonging useful life for many patients. Countless thousands have good reason to be thankful for cardiopulmonary resuscitation (CPR) and the numbers rise daily. Yet, in the wake of this advance, a small but important shadow of bizarre and distressing problems is present. These problems must be freely and openly addressed if we are to avoid criticism from others and from our own consciences.

Merely prolonging the process of dying

These apparent errors of judgement are caused by several factors. In a high proportion of cases, particularly those occurring outside hospital, the patient and his or her circumstances are unknown to the rescuer who may well not be competent to assess whether resuscitation is appropriate. Sadly, through lack of communication, this state of affairs also occurs from time to time in hospital practice. A junior ward nurse, unless explicitly instructed not to do so, feels, not unreasonably, obliged to call the resuscitation team to any patient with cardiorespiratory arrest. The nurse is not qualified to certify death. The team is often unaware of the patient's condition and prognosis and, because of the urgency of the situation, it begins treatment first and asks questions afterwards.

Ideally, resuscitation should be attempted only in patients who have a high chance of successful revival for a comfortable and contented existence. A study of published reports containing the results of series of resuscitation attempts shows that this ideal is far from being attained.

In retrospect, clearly in many cases the decision not to resuscitate could have been made before the event. As the number of deaths in hospital always exceeds the number of calls for resuscitation, a decision not to resuscitate is clearly being made. This situation does need improving.

The matter has been addressed by national authorities in the United States, by the European Resuscitation Council, and by the Resuscitation Council (UK) in their *Advanced Life Support Manual* (1998) and the joint manual with the European Resuscitation Council in 2001. Clearly, national differences exist that are dictated by legal, economic, religious, and social variables, but it is apparent that non-coercive guidelines can be set out to reduce the number of futile resuscitation attempts and to offer advice as to when resuscitation should be discontinued in the patient who does not respond.

The concept, from Australia, of the Medical Emergency Team (MET) that advocates a proactive role seems to offer a further way forward. Junior doctors and nurses are at liberty to call the team if a patient deteriorates in the general wards.

Selection of patients "not for resuscitation"
Two settings may be envisaged when the patients should not be resuscitated:

- The unexpected cardiorespiratory arrest with no other obvious underlying disease. In this situation resuscitation should be attempted without question or delay

---

Situations in which resuscitation is inappropriate

- Resuscitation attempts in the mortally ill do not enhance the dignity and serenity that we hope for our relatives and ourselves when we die
- All too often resuscitation is begun in patients already destined for life as cardiac or respiratory cripples or who are suffering the terminal misery of untreatable cancer
- From time to time, but fortunately rarely, resuscitation efforts may help to create the ultimate tragedy, the persistent vegetative state, because the heart is more tolerant than the brain to the insult of hypoxia

---

Survival rates after resuscitation

- The survival rates to discharge from hospital are 14-21%
- In each of these reports a substantial number, usually about 50-60%, failed to respond to the initial resuscitation attempts
- In many of these, particularly the younger patients, the effort was clearly justified initially
- The cause of the arrest was apparently myocardial ischaemia and the outcome cannot be confidently predicted in any individual patient
- Some of the papers, however, drew attention to the large proportion of patients in whom resuscitative efforts were inappropriate and unjustified; in one there was an incidence of 25% of patients in whom resuscitation merely prolonged the process of dying

---

Role of the MET

- Evaluate the patient's condition
- Advise on therapy
- Transfer to a critical care unit, usually in consultation with the doctor in charge of the patient
- In some situations recommend that to start resuscitation would be inappropriate

---

- Cardiorespiratory arrest in a patient with serious underlying disease. Patients in this group should be assessed beforehand as to whether a resuscitation attempt is considered appropriate.

The decision not to resuscitate revolves around many factors: the patient's own wishes, which may include a "living will," the patient's prognosis both immediate and long term, the views of relatives and friends, who may be reporting the known wishes of a patient who cannot communicate, and the patient's perceived ability to cope with disablement in the environment for which he or she is destined. Experience has shown that the "living will" often cannot be relied upon. The patient may have a change of mind when faced directly with death or may have envisaged death in different circumstances. The decision should not revolve around doctor pride.

Decisions on whether to resuscitate are generally made about each patient in the environment of close clinical supervision, which is prevalent in critical care units, and the decision is then communicated to the resident medical and nursing staff. In the general wards, however, the potential for cardiac arrest in specific patients may not actually be considered and inappropriate resuscitation occurs by default. Staff are reluctant to label a mentally alert patient, who is nevertheless terminally ill, "not for resuscitation." Sadly, doctors often refuse to acknowledge that the patient has reached end-stage disease, perhaps because they have spent so much time and effort in treating them. Some doctors, having spent their career in hospital practice, cannot comprehend the difficulties for the severely disabled of an existence without adequate help in a poor and miserable social environment. In addition, other doctors fear medicolegal sanctions if they put their name to an instruction not to resuscitate.

Fortunately, the climate of opinion is changing, and few members of the public or the profession now disagree with the concept of selecting patients deemed not suitable for resuscitation. The introduction of the MET may put the selection on a more experienced and scientific footing.

The final decision maker should be the senior doctor in charge of the patient's management. That senior doctor, however, will usually want to take cognisance of the opinions and wishes of the patient and the relatives and the views of the junior doctors, family practitioner, the MET if available, and nurses who have cared for the patient before arriving at a decision.

Once the decision not to resuscitate has been made, it should be clearly communicated to the medical and nursing staff on duty and recorded in the patient's notes. Because circumstances may change, the decision must be reviewed at intervals that may range from a few hours to weeks depending on the stability of the patient's condition.

A hospital ethical resuscitation policy

"Do not resuscitate" policies have been introduced in Canada and the United States. They tend to be very formal affairs with a strict protocol to be followed.

Nevertheless, to minimise tragedies and to improve success rates associated with resuscitation, it is helpful to establish an agreed non-coercive hospital ethical policy based on the principle of "resuscitation for all except when contraindicated." The promulgation of such guidelines serves as a reminder that the decision must be faced and made.

A hospital ethical resuscitation policy should contain the following guidelines:

- The decision not to resuscitate should be made by a senior doctor who should consult others as appropriate

---

> A 32 year old woman was admitted in a quadriplegic state due to a spinal injury incurred when she had thrown herself from the Clifton Suspension Bridge. She had made 18 previous attempts at suicide over the previous five years, sometimes by taking an overdose of tablets of various kinds and sometimes by cutting her wrists. She had been injecting herself with heroin for the past seven years and had no close relationship with her family and no close friends. During her stay of two days in the intensive care unit she developed pneumonia and died. A conscious decision not to provide artificial ventilation and resuscitation had been made beforehand

---

> A 62 year old woman had a cardiac arrest in a thoracic ward two days after undergoing pneumonectomy for resectable lung cancer. Her remaining lung was clearly fibrotic and malfunctioning, and her cardiac arrest was probably hypoxic and hypercarbic in origin. Because no instructions had been given to the contrary, she was resuscitated by the hospital resuscitation team and spontaneous cardiac rhythm restored after 20 minutes. She required continuous artificial ventilation and was unconscious for a week. Over the following six weeks she gradually regained consciousness but could not be weaned from the ventilator. She was tetraplegic, presumably as a result of spinal cord damage from hypoxia, but regained some weak finger movements over two months. At three months her improvement had tailed off, and she was virtually paralysed in all four limbs and dependent on the ventilator. She died five months after the cardiac arrest. She was supported throughout the illness by her devoted and intelligent husband, who left his work to be with her and continued to hope for a spontaneous cure until very near the end

---

Guidelines approved by the medical staff committee at Frenchay Hospital, Bristol

There can be no rules; every patient must be considered individually and this decision should be reviewed as appropriate—this may be on a weekly, daily, or hourly basis. The decision should be made before it is needed and in many patients this will be on admission.

The decision "Do not resuscitate" is absolutely compatible with continuing maximum therapeutic and nursing care.

- Where the patient is competent (that is, mentally fit and conscious), the decision "DO NOT RESUSCITATE" should be discussed where possible with the patient. This will not always be appropriate but, particularly in those patients with a slow progressive deterioration, it is important to consider it
- If the patient is not competent to make such decisions, the appropriate family members should be consulted
- Factors that may influence the decision to be made should include:
  - quality of life before this illness (highly subjective and only truly known to the patient himself)
  - expected quality of life (medical and social) assuming recovery from this particular illness
  - likelihood of resuscitation being successful.

The decision to "DO NOT RESUSCITATE" should be recorded clearly in medical and nursing notes, signed, and dated, and should be reviewed at appropriate intervals.

The above guidelines have been in use for the past 16 years and during this period no medical or nursing staff have objected to their use. However, experience has shown that continual reminders to the medical and nursing staff to address the questions in relevant cases are required

- The decision should be communicated to medical and nursing staff, recorded in the patient's notes, and reviewed at appropriate intervals
- The decision should be shared with the patient's relatives except in a few cases in which this would be inappropriate.

Other appropriate treatment and care should be continued.

Termination of resuscitation attempts

If resuscitation does not result in a relatively early return of spontaneous circulation then one of two options must be considered:

- Termination of further resuscitation efforts
- Support of the circulation by mechanical means, such as cardiac pacing, balloon pumping, or cardiopulmonary bypass.

The decision to terminate resuscitative efforts will depend on a number of factors discussed below.

The environment and access to emergency medical services

Cardiac arrest occurring in remote sites when access to emergency medical services (EMS) is impossible or very delayed is not associated with a favourable outcome.

Interval between onset of arrest and application of basic life support

This is crucial in determining whether the outcome will include intact neurological function. Generally speaking, if the interval is greater than five minutes then the prognosis is poor unless mitigating factors, such as hypothermia or previous sedative drug intake, are present. Children also tend to be more tolerant of delay.

Interval between basic life support and the application of advanced life support measures

Survival is rare if defibrillation and/or drug therapy is unavailable within 30 minutes of cardiac arrest. Each patient must be judged on individual merit, taking into account evidence of cardiac death, cerebral damage, and the ultimate prognosis.

Potential prognosis and underlying disease process

Resuscitation should be abandoned early in patients with a poor ultimate prognosis and end-stage disease. Prolonged attempts in such patients are rarely successful and are associated with a high incidence of cerebral damage.

Drug intake before cardiac arrest

Sedative, hypnotic, or narcotic drugs taken before cardiac arrest also provide a degree of cerebral protection against the effects of hypoxia and resuscitative efforts should be prolonged accordingly.

Remediable precipitating factors

Resuscitation should continue while the potentially remediable conditions giving rise to the arrest are treated. Such conditions include tension pneumothorax and cardiac tamponade. The outcome after cardiac arrest due to haemorrhagic hypovolaemia is notoriously poor. Factors to be taken into account include the immediate availability of very skilled surgery and very rapid transfusion facilities. Even under optimal conditions survival rates are poor and early termination of resuscitation is generally indicated if bleeding cannot be immediately controlled.

Evidence of cardiac death

Persistent ventricular fibrillation should be actively treated until established asystole or electromechanical dissociation (pulseless electrical activity) supervenes. Patients with asystole who are unresponsive to adrenaline (epinephrine) and fluid replacement are unlikely to survive except in extenuating circumstances. Resuscitation should be abandoned after 15 minutes

Evidence of cerebral damage

Persistent fixed and dilated pupils, unrelated to previous drug therapy, are usually, but not invariably, an indication of serious cerebral damage, and consideration should be given to abandoning resuscitation in the absence of mitigating factors. If a measurement system is in place, intracranial pressure values greater than 30 mmHg are a poor prognostic sign

Age

Age in itself has less effect on outcome than the underlying disease process or the presenting cardiac rhythm. Nevertheless, patients in their 70s and 80s do not have good survival rates compared with their younger fellow citizens generally because of underlying disease, and earlier curtailment of resuscitative efforts is indicated. By contrast, young children, on occasion, seem to be tolerant of hypoxia and resuscitation should be continued for longer than in adults

Temperature

Hypothermia confers protection against the effects of hypoxia. Resuscitation efforts should be continued for much longer in hypothermic than in normothermic patients; situations have been reported of survival with good neurological function after more than 45 minutes submersion in water. Resuscitation should be continued in hypothermic patients during active rewarming using cardiopulmonary bypass if available and appropriate (see Chapter 15)

Other ethical problems arising in relation to resuscitation

A number of other unsolved ethical problems do arise in relation to resuscitation, which need to be addressed.

The diagnosis of death

Traditionally, and in most countries, death is pronounced by medical practitioners. However, the question arises as to the wisdom and practicality of death being determined in some cases by non-medical healthcare professionals, such as nurses and ambulance personnel.

The recognition (or validation) of death and formal certification are profoundly different. Formal certification must, by law, be undertaken by a registered medical practitioner, and this requirement will not change. Nevertheless, it is possible to identify patients in whom survival is very unlikely and when resuscitation would be both futile and distressing for relatives, friends, and healthcare personnel, and situations in which time and resources would be wasted in undertaking such measures. In such cases it has been proposed that the recognition of death may be undertaken by someone other than a registered medical practitioner, such as a trained ambulance paramedic or technician. In introducing such a proposal, it is essential to ensure that death is not erroneously diagnosed and a potential survivor is denied resuscitation.

To avoid such an error, clear and simple guidelines have been drawn up in the United Kingdom by the Joint Royal Colleges Ambulance Liaison Committee identifying conditions unequivocally associated with death and those in which an electrocardiogram (ECG) will assist the diagnosis. In addition, a further group of patients with terminal illness should not be resuscitated when the wishes of the patient and doctor have been made clear.

No instances have been recorded of patients surviving with the conditions listed in group A, nor of adults who have been submersed for over three hours. Authorities are agreed that it is totally inappropriate to commence resuscitation in these circumstances. The futility of CPR in patients with mortal trauma has been highlighted in several publications. The concept of a "Do Not Resuscitate" policy has received international support for patients with terminal illness whose condition has been recently reviewed by the family doctor, in consultation with the relatives and patient where appropriate. A study of 1461 patients found that when persistent ventricular fibrillation was excluded, all survivors had a return of spontaneous circulation within 20 minutes. No patient survived with asystole lasting longer than this time. In another group of 1068 patients who experienced out-of-hospital cardiac arrest, only three survived among those who were transported to hospital with ongoing CPR. Those three survivors were discharged from hospital with moderate to severe cerebral disability. These findings support the proposal that death may be recognised in normothermic patients who have had a period of asystole lasting at least 15 minutes.

It has been suggested that resuscitation attempts should be abandoned in patients with cardiac arrest in whom the time of collapse to the arrival of ambulance personnel exceeds 15 minutes, provided that no attempt at CPR has been made in that time interval and the ECG has shown an unshockable rhythm. This recommendation is supported by a review of 414 patients who had not received any CPR in the 15 or more minutes to ambulance arrival. No patient survived who had a non-shockable rhythm when the first ECG was recorded. This resulted in an algorithm for ambulance personnel

Other resuscitation procedures

Use of cardiac pacing
- Cardiac pacing (internal or transthoracic) has little application in cardiac arrest. Pacing should be reserved for those patients with residual P wave activity or with very slow rhythms (see Chapter 17)

Balloon pump and cardiopulmonary bypass
- Clearly, use of this equipment depends on the immediate availability of the apparatus and skilled staff to operate it. Such intervention should be reserved for patients with a potentially good prognosis—for example cases of hypothermia, drug overdose, and those with conditions amenable to immediate cardiac, thoracic, or abdominal surgery

---

Extract of Joint Royal Colleges Ambulance Liaison Committee Guidelines

Group A—Conditions unequivocally associated with death
- Decapitation
- Massive cranial and cerebral destruction
- Hemicorporectomy (or similar massive injury)
- Decomposition
- Incineration
- Rigor mortis
- Fetal maceration

In these groups, death can be recognised by the clinical confirmation of cardiac arrest

Group B—Conditions requiring ECG evidence of asystole
- Submersion for more than three hours in adults over 18 years of age, with or without hypothermia
- Continuous asystole, despite cardiopulmonary resuscitation (CPR), for more than 20 minutes in a normothermic patient
- Patients who have received no resuscitation for at least 15 minutes after collapse and who have no pulse or respiratory effort on arrival of the ambulance personnel

Timings must be accurate
In all these cases, the ECG record must be free from artefact and show asystole. There must be no positive history of sedative, hypnotic, anxiolytic, opiate, or anaesthetic drugs in the preceding 24 hours

Group C—Terminal illness
Cases of terminal illness when the doctor has given clear instructions that the patient is not for resuscitation

---

Issues in training

Use of the recently dead for practical skills training
Opportunities for hands-on training in the practical skills required for resuscitation are limited. It is clear that tracheal intubation cannot be taught to everyone attending a cardiac arrest. Although the laryngeal mask may offer an alternative option for airway management in the short term, the introduction of that device on a widespread scale into anaesthetic practice has, in itself, reduced the opportunities for training in the anaesthetic room. Manikin training offers an alternative, but most would agree that training on patients is required to amplify manikin experience. Training in tracheal intubation on the recently dead has engendered a sharp debate and, although supported by some doctors, has met with strong opposition from members of the nursing profession. Informed consent is difficult to obtain at the sensitive and emotional time of bereavement, and approaches to relatives may be construed as coercion. Proceeding without consent may be considered as assault.

The dilemma does not stop with tracheal intubation, and other techniques, such as fibre optic intubation, central venous access, surgical cut-down venous access, chest drain insertion, and surgical cricothyrotomy, should be considered.

encountering death in these conditions, which has been accepted by the Professional Advisory Group of the Scottish Ambulance Service and the Central Legal Office to the Scottish Office Health Department.

The validity of the proposed guidelines depends on the accurate diagnosis being cardiac arrest within the first 15 or so minutes of the "collapse." As cardiac arrest might not, in fact, occur at the time of the initial collapse, the period of unsupported arrest could be less—perhaps much less—than 15 minutes. In these circumstances, resuscitation could possibly still be successful. When the 15 minute asystole guideline has been used in the United States, however, this concern has proved to be unfounded.

Whether or not these guidelines are followed, it is important that it is made clear what local arrangements should be followed by ambulance personnel once they have made a diagnosis of death. These must be disseminated throughout the service and to all other concerned groups.

Legal aspects

Doctors, nurses, and paramedical staff functioning in their official capacity have an obligation to perform CPR when medically indicated and in the absence of a "Do Not Resuscitate" decision.

Many countries apply "Good Samaritan" laws in relation to CPR to protect lay rescuers acting in good faith, provided they are not guilty of gross negligence. In other countries the law may not be specifically written down but the "Good Samaritan" principle is applied by the judiciary. Such arrangements are essential for the creation and continuance of community and hospital CPR policies. At the time of writing, the author does not know of any case in which a lay person who has made a reasonable attempt at CPR has been successfully sued. Similar protection applies to teachers and trainers of citizen CPR programmes.

Healthcare professionals performing CPR outside their place of work and acting as bystander citizens are expected to perform basic CPR within the limitations of the environment and facilities available to them.

When acting in an official capacity, healthcare professionals are expected to be able to perform basic life support, and all doctors are expected additionally to provide the major elements of advanced life support, including airway management, ventilation with oxygen, defibrillation, intravenous cannulation, and appropriate drug therapy. Hospitals are expected to provide the appropriate resuscitation equipment and facilities. With increasing expectation of higher standards it is likely that these requirements will extend to family medical and dental practices; leisure, sports, and travel centres; trains; airplanes; ships; and major workplaces in the future.

The status of a "Do Not Resuscitate" policy is rarely defined precisely in the legislature of most European countries. The majority of the judiciary, however, accept in practice that a decision not to resuscitate has been carefully arrived at and is based on the guidelines outlined above.

Conclusion

Modern medicine brings problems and ethical dilemmas. Public expectations have changed and will continue to change. Increasingly, doctors' actions are questioned in the media and in the courts of law. We need to formulate answers and be more open with the public to explain how our actions are related entirely to their wellbeing. Only in this way will we keep in tune with society and practise the science of resuscitation with art and compassion.

The involvement of relatives and close friends

Bystanders should be encouraged to undertake immediate basic life support in the event of cardiorespiratory arrest. In many cases the bystander will be a close relative. Traditionally, relatives have been escorted away from the victim when the healthcare professionals arrive. However, it is clear that some relatives do not wish to be isolated from their loved one at this time and are deeply hurt if this is enforced. The Resuscitation Council (UK) has confirmed the need to identify and respect relatives' wishes to remain with the victim. Clearly, care and consideration of the relative in these stressful situations become of increasing concern as the invasive nature of the resuscitation attempt escalates from basic life support, to defibrillation and venous access, and perhaps to chest drainage, cricothyrotomy, and even open chest cardiac massage

Further reading

- Adams S, Whitlock M, Higgs R, Bloomfield P, Baskett PJF. Should relatives be allowed to watch resuscitation? *BMJ* 1994;308:1689.
- American Heart Association, Emergency Cardiac Care Committee. Baskett PJF. Ethics in cardiopulmonary resuscitation. *Resuscitation* 1993;25:1-8.
- Bonnin MJ, Pepe PE, Kimball KT, Clark PS. Distinct criteria for termination of resuscitation in the out of hospital setting. *JAMA* 1993;270:1457-62.
- Bossaert L. Ethical issues in resuscitation. In: Vincent JL, ed. *Yearbook of intensive care and emergency medicine.* New York: Springer Verlag, 1994.
- Centers for Disease Control. Update: universal precautions for prevention of transmission of human immunodeficiency virus, hepatitis B virus and other blood borne pathogens in health care-settings. *Morbid Mortal Wkly Rep* 1988;37:377-88.
- Royal College of Nursing, British Medical Association, Resuscitation Council (UK). Cardiopulmonary resuscitation—a statement from the Royal College of Nursing, the British Medical Association and the Resuscitation Council (UK), March 1993.
- Guidelines for cardiopulmonary resuscitation and emergency cardiac care. Ethical considerations in resuscitation. *JAMA* 1992;268:2282-8.
- International guidelines 2000 for cardiopulmonary resuscitation and emergency cardiac care—an international consensus on science. *Resuscitation* 2000;46:17-28.
- Gwinnutt CL, Columb M, Harris R. Outcome after cardiac arrest in adults in UK hospitals: effect of the 1997 guidelines. *Resuscitation* 2000;47:125-35.
- Hillman K, Parr M, Flabouris A, Bishop G, Stewart A. Redefining in hospital resuscitation—the concept of the Medical Emergency Team. *Resuscitation* 2001;48:102-10.
- Holmberg S, Ekstrom L. Ethics and practicalities of resuscitation. *Resuscitation* 1992;24:239-44.
- Joint Royal Colleges Ambulance Liaison Committee. *Newsletter 1996 and 2001.* Royal College of Physicians, London.
- Kellerman AL, Hackman BB, Somes G. Predicting the outcome of unsuccessful prehospital advanced cardiac life support. *JAMA* 1993;270:1433-6.
- Marsden AK, Ng GA, Dalziel K, Cobbe SM. When is it futile for ambulance personnel to initiate cardiopulmonary resuscitation? *BMJ* 1995;311:49-51.
- Resuscitation Council UK. *Advanced life support manual.* London: Resuscitation Council UK, 1998 and 2001.
- Parr MJA, Hadfield JH, Flabouris A, Bishop G, Hillman K. The Medical Emergency Team: 12 month analysis of reasons for activation, immediate outcome and not-for-resuscitation orders. *Resuscitation* 2001;50:39-44.

Index

Page numbers in **bold** type refer to figures; those in *italic* refer to tables or boxed material.

Index

Index

The complete ABC series

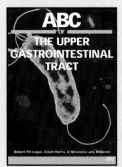

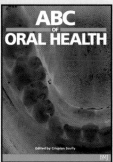

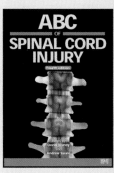

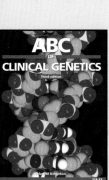

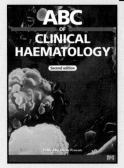